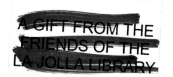

A
Beautiful
New
 # You

OTHER BOOKS BY LAURA DuPRIEST

Natural Beauty: Pamper Yourself With Salon Secrets at Home

A
Beautiful
New
You

LAURA DuPRIEST

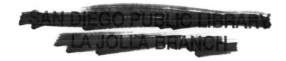
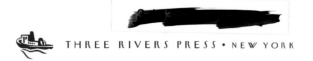
THREE RIVERS PRESS • NEW YORK

Published in the United States by Three Rivers Press, an imprint of the
Crown Publishing Group, a division of Random House, Inc., New York.
www.crownpublishing.com

Three Rivers Press and the Tugboat design are registered trademarks of Random House, Inc.

Library of Congress Cataloging-in-Publication Data

DuPriest, Laura.
A beautiful new you : inspiration and practical advice to transform your looks and your life—
a total makeover without cosmetic surgery / Laura DuPriest.
1. Beauty, Personal.   2. Women—Health and hygiene.   I. Title.
RA778.D935   2005
646.7'042—dc22   2004021216

ISBN 1-4000-5476-1

Printed in the United States of America

Design by Helene Berinsky

10   9   8   7   6   5   4   3   2   1

First Edition

For my father and mother,
who gave me my ruby slippers
and taught me that I could
achieve anything I set out
to accomplish.

ACKNOWLEDGMENTS

An extraordinary team of compassionate people that believed in me and this rewarding project helped to create this book. It is my privilege and an honor to express my deepest gratitude to each and every one of them for bringing this vital message to women.

First and foremost, I would like to thank my clients for seeking to improve their lives with a sense of pride in themselves. I feel blessed to be a part of your transformations, your dreams, your successes, and most important, your lives. Each and every one of you is precious.

I will never forget the day that I showed my "before" photo to Charlie Benard, CEO of Laura DuPriest LLC. He insisted with his usual honesty and conviction that I tell my story. Charlie's insight and determination were the cornerstone of this inspirational book. Thank you, Charlie, for your countless hours of hard work, creative instinct, and leadership and for establishing our incredible company. I would also like to extend my gratitude to Marc Cawdrey, chief marketing officer, for his talent, experience, and marketing expertise, and to Jason Dunlop, vice president of finance, for the myriad details he so gracefully masters.

A boatload of appreciation for the dynamic staff at Three Rivers Press steered by editor Becky Cabaza. I am grateful to Becky for her wisdom and for believing that this was much more than a beauty book, and I feel lucky to have worked with her and her team. Thank you to Orly Trieber for her constant guidance and input and to the team at Three Rivers Press: Susan Westendorf, Laura Duffy, Lauren Dong, Laurie McGee, and Helene Berinsky. Working with all of you was great fun.

Thank you to Jennifer Basey Sander for her kind introduction to Charlie Benard, thus creating the beginning of this big adventure. Jennifer, I owe you!

Over three years ago, my friend Jennifer Smith asked me try a makeover on the Midday News she coanchored with Dan Elliott at News10, the ABC affiliate in Sacramento. Since then, News10 has presented nearly two hundred beautiful transformations for women of all ages. I am so appreciative to Russell Postell, president/general manager and the entire team at News10 for dramatically changing the lives of so many people. Thank you Margaret Mohr, marketing director; Ron Comings, news director; Kristi Gordon, Midday producer (bless you, Kristi, for your patience and kindness) and all the Midday crew: Chris Garvey, Steve Cornelius, Ed Hernandez, Claudia Johnson, Brian Plumb, Greg Branche, Dennis Eastman, Connie Hamataka, Joe Lee, Gary Miles, Kelly Olson, Julie Middleburg, Darrell Britt, Paula Blair, Don Bailey, Akiko Yanagi, Kate Moore, Daniel McChesney, Bob Montgomery, Elizabeth Bishop, Kevin Williams, Christine Huber, Dennis Allen, and D'arcy Ward. To Jennifer Smith, who started all of this, my deepest thanks, for I have learned so much from your grace and talent. To Dan Elliott, you have inspired me with your humor and natural style; Monday mornings are more fun because of you. Continued thanks to all the on-camera talent whom I have had the pleasure to work beside: Monica Woods, Melissa Crowley, Alicia Malaby, J. D. Maher, Darla Givens, Dana Howard, and Jonathan Mumm.

Putting the processes of personal transformation down on paper was not easy. I am deeply grateful to Caroline Benard for her tremendous contribution in making this book a reality. Caroline spent hours and hours right by my side handling just about everything from interviews to art direction, from formatting to editing. I couldn't have produced these inspirational pages without her.

Writing a book while managing a business and holding down the fort with two children was the greatest challenge of my life. The person who kept me sane with his love, support, and skilled writing assistance was my best friend for life, Dan Gray. I am overwhelmed with appreciation for his personal dedication and enthusiasm in bringing this book to women. Thank you for the many hours of interviewing, researching, and assisting my writing and editing. Most important, thank you for gentle nudges to keep going and for fueling my heart.

There is a lot of talent from dynamic artists bound together in these pages. My admiration and gratitude goes out to my salon staff for their makeover skills and undying support. Thank you, Michelle Camacho, Cecelia Addun-Powell, Natalia Titerenko, Amy Davis, Corrie Heiman, Christine Galindo, Anne Zavala, Tracy Fowler, Monica Camacho, Sara Hisey, Maria Fernandez, Mason Munson, Stacy Brownson, and Lucy Arteaga. The photographs in this book feature the work of your talented hands and artistic eyes.

A special hug and a squeeze for Tara Weyand. Thank you for your loving embrace of friendship and continual support. You fueled me with your goodness and encouragement.

A thousand kisses for Tony and Johnny, my incredible sons for every day that they showed me what life is all about. Leaving Mom alone to write every day was not easy, but they respectfully did it. They listened to my rough drafts and even made corrections and suggestions. I love you guys!

I would like to give artistic kudos to Bryan Kwong, who came to my aid during a holiday weekend to illustrate the makeup lessons, and to Jeff Markowitz for his patience and keen eye photographing our makeovers.

To Jeff Lujan, my special friend, bless you for your photographic talent and for making this retired model feel great in front of the camera again. Jeff, it's easy to smile when you're behind the lens.

My transformation was accomplished initially because of a huge weight loss. I will be eternally grateful to Larry Gury, Russ Kuhn, and the entire team of employees at the California Family Fitness Centers. Your brilliant idea to cultivate family fitness has changed the lives of so many people. My children and I will always remember the fun-filled hours spending time together while enjoying health and fitness. Special thanks to Nick Gury, Jeremy Schulz, Daniel Kerian, and Norvell Peoples. God bless all of you!

I am privileged to know some incredible business associates who are also my good friends. Thank you for pitching in to help create this book. To Randy Paragary and Danny Sullivan for letting us take over K-bar for our photo shoots. To Carol Greenberg at The Learning Exchange for suggesting that I spread the word and teach! To Ed Dunbar and Ann Huntley at Café Dolce for your moral support and delicious food you prepare for my fitness eating. Special thanks as well to Greg Virga, Tony Babcock, and the entire staff at Jack's Urban Eats in Sacramento for the healthy evening meals and to David Berkley and staff for the splendid afternoon snacks. I lost most of my seventy-five pounds somewhere in your restaurants!

For their special contributions of support, my heartfelt thanks to Eric Swanson, my Web designer, Gunter Stannius, Tony Walker, Cheryl Danforth, Doug Link, Gary Pannullo, John Harris, Cary Nosler, Mishal Lamont, Charlotte Barkman, Mary Gomes, Corey Egel, Janice Watkins, Linda DuPriest, Kathleen Finnerty, Ed Wright, and Bill Stall.

Lastly, one of the most important people of my life, my dear friend Craig Harris, who started all of this when he created Natural Beauty for Public Television. His idea to bring natural cosmetic and beauty solutions to women was nominated for an Emmy Award and then a book. Not long after *Natural Beauty, Pamper Yourself With Salon Secrets at Home* was published, Craig encouraged me to write again. I told him about my motivational inspiration, my ruby slippers. He said, "Write it." I dedicate my ruby slippers to you, Craig. Thank you for keeping me on the path and for your spiritual guidance.

CONTENTS

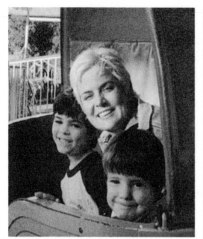

Laura DuPriest before

INTRODUCING THE BEAUTIFUL NEW YOU

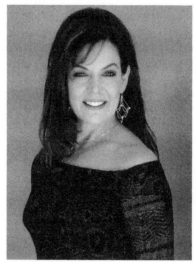

Laura DuPriest after

This is a book about hope. Within these pages, I promise to give you hope and the power to make your life better. What do I mean by better? Just to look better? Perhaps that is why you bought this book, but in addition to learning how to improve your appearance, you will come to understand that looking and feeling better will dramatically change every aspect of your life!

How would you like to wake up tomorrow projecting confidence and radiance? It's time to give yourself permission to change, and I can help make that happen. What I am going to teach you comes from having experienced the glorious reality of a head-to-toe transformation that literally restored hope in my life. I am going to give that same hope to you.

Though I'm in the business of making people beautiful—including making people "over"—I first had to make over myself and experience the pain and joy of that journey before I could share the knowledge of radiant rebirth with others.

You may have picked up this book because, like thousands of other women, you suddenly found yourself in a place you didn't like—you no longer feel at your personal best. You may have even been wondering, "Where did I go? What happened to me? What happened to the attractive, confident person I once was?" Or perhaps you feel pretty good about yourself but just want a little help in the beauty department—without the intimidation and confusion that sometimes lurk behind a makeup counter or in a department store dressing room.

Your Makeover, Your Second Life

Second life? Yes. You see, your first life undoubtedly belonged to other people and other things: college, husband, children, job, and simply keeping up with the ordinary demands of life. Your second life belongs to you. I will show you in this book how to fall back in love with life and be an example to others. My pledge is to show you that the more you nurture yourself, the more energy you'll have for everyone in your world. By giving to yourself, I guarantee you'll have more strength to help those important people around you.

My personal story will be shared throughout this book because I believe that so many women have suffered the same frustration I experienced—trying to be all things to all people, but at the same time neglecting myself. I was convinced that taking care of myself was frivolous, that there wasn't time, that I was too tired or it didn't matter. But it *did* matter. Eventually, my "letting go" of myself showed on the outside, but it also was indicative of something more important crumbling on the inside, the erosion of my self-worth and then my self-esteem. Sound familiar? Well, don't panic or feel ashamed or hopeless. I promised you hope, and I will fulfill that promise. My mission is to share my knowledge and personal transformation experience with you and lead you down an exciting pathway to your own magical transformation.

This isn't a book about plastic surgery, but certainly that option is more and more of a possibility for an increasing number of women. Instead, I'd like you to focus on things about your appearance that you can change on your own, and you'd be surprised just how much power you have. This book won't make you five foot eleven if you are only five foot two, but after reading and using this book to transform your life, you will walk tall from the inside out. Your makeover will reach far beyond your reflection in the mirror. It will make over your attitude, your self-esteem, and your entire life.

How to Use This Book

A lot of critical information is presented in this book, but I realize that you may want to dive right in and take action immediately. That's great. I want you to begin experiencing your new life and renewed hope right away. Each chapter is a new step down the pathway leading to your transformation. In the beginning, I will help you make over your thinking and mentally prepare you for the physical changes you may want to make. In each chapter, you will meet amazing women just like you, who have successfully achieved real-life transformations that rekindled their optimism. They have agreed to share their stories in the hope that you may be inspired to embark on your own personal journey. At the end of each chapter there will be a new, easy-to-complete step in your **Makeover Action Plan.** Your Makeover Action Plan, or your MAP, will be your road map to guide you on your path to realistically and radically change your life for the better. You'll be asked to write down your thoughts and feelings, as well as chart your progress in beauty and exercise, and you can do so in the space provided, or in a separate journal or notebook. This way, you'll be able to look back at your journey to remind yourself of just how far you have come.

Some of you will want to read this entire book before setting your wheels in motion. Others may want to get right down to making instant changes. I encourage you to use this book the way you want to. Here's a quick guide on ways to get started.

I just want a little update on makeup and hair.
- Go directly to Step 5, "Your Beauty Revealed," and look over the real makeovers, see color insert, for inspiration.
- Read chapters 12 and 13 for step-by-step instructions.

I'm curious about makeovers, but I haven't decided if I need one or not.
- Skim over the entire book.
- Read chapter 4, "Imagine the All New You."
- Look over the real makeovers.
- Read the chapters in Step 5 for some great how-tos.
- Read the entire book if you need more help.

I always take care of myself but just need to get back in shape.
- Skim over the entire book.
- Read Step 4, "Your Mental Makeover."
- Read chapters 15 and 16 to jump-start you back into getting fit.
- Read Step 5, "Your Beauty Revealed," for inspiration and some great how-tos.
- Read the entire book if you need more help.

I have been neglecting myself for years, and I feel like a frump.
- Look at the real makeover photos for inspiration.
- Read the entire book with pencil in hand to start your new life.

Don't worry about how and when you'll accomplish your makeover. Some of the women in this book made instant changes in a day while others reshaped their bodies over a few months, some over a few years. What they all shared with me was the revelation that life was instantly more fulfilling for them simply by making the choice to do something for *them*.

I know that this book will teach you new and exciting ways to transform your appearance, but I also know from my experience and that of my makeover friends that it will change your life.

STEP ONE

Your Awakening

"Like anyone else, there are days when I feel beautiful and days when I don't. When I don't, I do something about it."

—CHERYL TIEGS

Your Epiphany

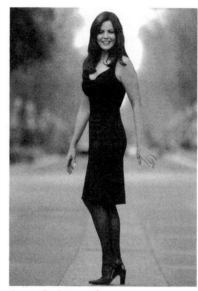

Laura DuPriest before

Laura DuPriest after

"Your life changes the moment you make a new, congruent, committed decision."

—ANTHONY ROBBINS

It was my son Tony's ninth birthday party and I remember feeling excited and a little giddy because I was giving the party at a local amusement park. The gathering was going to be small, just my immediate family and a few friends, so throwing on a pair of shorts and tennis shoes was an easy decision. As I pawed through my dresser drawers looking for my favorite comfy khakis, I smiled in anticipation of the time off from work to ride a roller coaster or Ferris wheel with my boys. I enthusiastically stepped into my shorts, pulled them up to button them. Looking down, I could clearly see the two-inch gap between the button and the buttonhole. Hmmmm. I pulled the waistband up higher, and sucked it in. With great determination and effort, I managed to secure the button and hoist the zipper up halfway. I heaved in a heavy sigh. My zipper had been flying at half-mast for the past few months. But I had a party to attend so I shook it off with my old standby thinking that the washer had caused the garment to shrink. Yeah, that was it. Next time I'll remember to wash with cold water! I grabbed a baggy sweatshirt and a jeans jacket to cover the gaping zipper and hurried off to celebrate.

My boys and I arrived at the park before the rest of the family in order to set the table and decorate. As I watched my two young sons pass out plates and cups, pride swelled up in me; I was impressed with their helpful nature and pleased that they were bright, polite, and handsome little boys. Soon, bits and pieces of my very large family trickled in, including my parents, Grandma and Grandpa. As my dad got closer I could see his frown and his stare just above my forehead. He was trying to size up the way he felt about my hair color. It was canary yellow. My natural color was a deep brown. I had just had it bleached at my salon, thinking that it would make me look chic, fashionable, and hip. The cut was new as well, very short and kind of spiky, another brainstorm of mine to make me look modern.

My father, being a very honest and passionate man, has no problem expressing himself. "What have you done to your hair, and why did you do it?" I felt as if I was in an *I Love Lucy* episode, only Ethel wasn't there to share the humiliation. "I decided to go blond!" I declared proudly. I looked from his scowl to my mom, hoping to get some encouragement or approval. She looked as if she was in pain, not knowing whether to soothe me by contradicting my father's opinion or to be honest and hurt my feelings. She took the diplomatic route, "It's a change . . . uh, something different!" Dad's scowl turned into a roll of the eyes. Again, I brushed off the sinking feeling of self-doubt and attributed the remarks to Dad being a fuddy-duddy. (Anyway, I thought, men like blond hair!)

The afternoon proved to be a blast as twelve wild kids scurried around the amusement park with nine parents in tow. Eventually we all ended up seated around a big table eating cake and ice cream. As I enjoyed my second serving of cake, I felt the eyes of one of my brothers upon me. I looked up to find him staring blankly at me. "What?" I asked. John shook his head and said, "I've never seen you fat; you don't even look like you." My brother is not a mean person so his comment didn't impact me at the moment. I just smiled and began cleaning up. Even with three strikes against me that day, I sluffed it off. To me, I was okay, fine, perfect. I had no clue about how I looked to my family or anyone else. I quite frankly was too busy to notice or focus on my reality. The only conclusion I arrived at was that my pants were too tight, especially after my cake feast. I made a mental note to shop the next day for some shorts that would fit. Perhaps I would choose a size larger so the washer wouldn't play that evil game with me again.

Tony's birthday party should have been an awakening for me because of the bombardment of negativity, but I had been perfecting the art of ignoring myself and making the best of things. For seven years, I'd been raising my children alone and devoting my days (and nights) to running my own business, focusing on making a living for my family, not the reflection I saw in the mirror. Deep down, I knew that reflection had undergone some dramatic and negative changes from head to toe, but I had become an expert at denial and self-neglect. Why should a frown from my dad, a negative comment from my brother, or a pair of tight shorts get me down? My standard MO was to simply ignore it and press on with life. Solve the problem. Buy new pants.

There was nothing on my agenda the following day, a Sunday, except to be a couch potato and shop for pants that fit. In the late afternoon, I headed out alone to the Target store a few blocks from my house. In the past, I would shop for 8's or 10's by holding the garments up to my waist and guessing if they would fit. (I despised trying on clothes in the fitting room.) After surfing the racks for some size 10 jeans, I quickly assessed that they were not even close to reaching across the front of my body. Next I tried 12's, then 14's. *Wow,* I thought to myself, *their sizes must be really screwed up!* I headed into the dressing room with the evil size 14 jeans. I grabbed the 12's as well . . . hoping . . . praying. Before I slipped out of my shorts, I made sure the curtain was completely closed, determined to keep secret what I was about to find out. Even before I could get the size 12 jeans up past my knees I knew it would be impossible to zip them up. I kicked them off and quickly tried on the 14's. The pressure of the denim on my thighs was almost as humiliating as the flattening of my beefy tush. I looked in the mirror and realized what my body actually looked like. Puffy, swollen, lumpy, and just plain old HUGE. Slowly I turned around, bent over slightly, and looked over my shoulder to get the real view of my backside. My neck got warm and I started to feel the panic. Swiftly, I scrambled out of the jeans as if they were on fire and left them in a heap on the floor. As I left the store I began comparing myself to all the other women who were strolling the aisles. Many of the others looked the same as me, plumpish and plain, some in sweats and baseball caps. That didn't make me feel any better. They made me see more clearly what I looked like. My pace quickened as I headed for my car, and it was as if someone or something was chasing or attacking me. The hot feeling at the back of my neck turned into a full body sweat. I was having a panic attack. Fear and dread washed over me in a flood. I pointed the car toward the freeway and headed to my parents' house. I would seek comfort and approval from my mom.

The thirty-minute drive out to my folks' house was agonizing. I bit my lower lip and stole glances at myself in the rearview mirror. My brother's words from the day before haunted me—he didn't recognize me anymore. The mirror reflected the image of my chubby face, my double chin, and my freaky-looking haircut. My complexion appeared dull and colorless. My eye color used to be a brilliant blue. Now, it was a faded gray. I looked completely washed out because of the peculiar, baby-chick-yellow hair color. My brother was right. I didn't look like myself. Not at all.

"Stop looking in the mirror," I told myself and pressed on. I needed my mom. My mother is the sweetest person in the world. Just being around her makes people feel good. I didn't forewarn her that I was coming; I just showed up in her kitchen. As she turned to me I asked, "Mom, do I look like a size 14?" (I didn't really want the truth; I just wanted her to make me feel better.) Her hesitation was all the information I needed. She gazed down from my face to my body and back up again. "Yes, sweetie, you do." It was at that moment, I had my epiphany. I gave my mom a hug and headed home. It was a long, quiet drive.

Your Epiphany

If you are like me, you may not have realized how far you slipped off the beauty path until you get back on track to the radiant beauty you used to be. It took trying to squeeze into a pair of tight jeans to snap me into reality. Prior to that day, I was blazing through life too busy to look at what I was presenting to the world. Perhaps you have already had your "tight jeans" moment. Or you developed a roll of film and were aghast at what you saw. Perhaps you've received a comment or nudge from your family and maybe the remarks caused you to feel hurt. What was your epiphany?

Many women I have counseled experienced a panic attack based on a moment or event such as I did. The word *epiphany* comes from the Greek word *epiphaneia*, "appearance." A realization. An acute awareness. The epiphany marks the point of no return. Enough is enough. Experiencing your epiphany may have taken place in a blink of an eye, or it may have involved a slower process of realization. In either case, recognizing or experiencing this pivotal moment can swiftly turn into motivation.

COLLEEN'S STORY

Colleen Morgan remembers her epiphany, the exact moment she realized she *had* to change her life. She and her family were watching

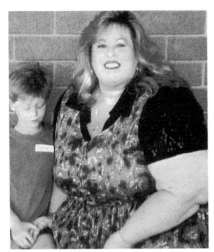

Colleen Morgan before

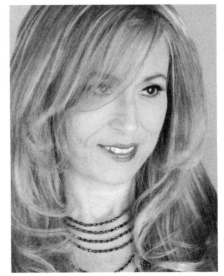

Colleen Morgan after

their video of Easter morning. Looking at herself on the TV screen gave Colleen a perspective of how others viewed her. Colleen saw a 475-pound woman who did not match her self-image. She didn't feel that big. But that picture was burned into her mind, and for two days she felt unhappy and ashamed. On the third day she was tired of feeling sorry for herself and decided to take action. Colleen met with a personal trainer and they developed a plan: "I was a woman who needed a change, and I changed my life for the better."

The change took Colleen from the couch where she faithfully watched soap operas every day to a swimming pool where she faithfully exercised three days a week, sometimes five hours a day. As large as Colleen was, walking without the aid of a swimming pool was difficult. She began walking laps in the pool. As the pounds started to melt she advanced to swimming laps and water aerobics. Colleen's confidence was being restored as she shed about five pounds a week during the first few months of working out.

Over a seven-year period Colleen lost 230 pounds. "I'm very

happy. I wish I would have done this earlier in my life," Colleen told me. Exercise and diet were now priorities—remarkable commitments from a woman who was afraid to go out of the house after her first child was born. Feeling out of shape after a pregnancy, Colleen found comfort in food. After a second child there was more weight gain. Overcoming her fear of change, this proud mother is now a role model for her children. "Both of my boys are proud of me. My oldest even works out with me at the gym, and my youngest can't wait until he is old enough to work out with Mom. I'm very proud that I am a healthy role model for my children," Colleen says with a big smile.

Dramatic changes occurred in her social life. To avoid seeing the stares of others, the old Colleen would keep her head down during her rare shopping trips.

The new Colleen feels no embarrassment as she shops for clothes with girlfriends once a week. Head held high and looking me directly in the eye she beams, "I am more confident and more outgoing and not afraid to live my life anymore. My husband brags about me. My message to anyone who reads this book is that you've got to change everything. It is a total lifestyle change."

Enjoying a more shapely figure at age forty, Colleen looks and feels better than she did in her twenties. And now she has set new goals. "I accomplished something I thought I could not do. I enter walk-a-thons now and in each one I have improved my finish time. Now my goal is to compete in a triathlon."

Colleen's message is to change everything. Like Colleen, you may be fed up with your current situation and are prepared to completely alter your lifestyle. On the other hand, changing just one aspect of your life—such as eating healthier food or taking one hour a day to go to the gym—may be the key. It could be something very simple, like spending a half hour uninterrupted doing your hair or makeup. Whatever the case, I bet something stirred inside you that prompted you to consider changing *something*. I will continue to refer to that pivotal moment as *your epiphany*.

When your epiphany happens, one of the most important things that occurs is that you are suddenly willing to put your own needs at the same level as the demands of your job, or the needs of your mate or children. You realize that it's okay to devote time to yourself, even though it might feel selfish. It's not. It is one of the most loving things you can do for yourself and for everyone who loves you. So many women come into my salon and spa and say things like, "My husband doesn't want me to cut my hair" or "I don't have the time to fix myself up" or "It's frivolous to spend the time and money on myself." These women haven't realized their self-worth. They haven't decided that they are valuable enough to make the effort to change. The reality, however, is that they obviously *want* to look terrific; otherwise they would not have made an appointment.

If you are reluctant to value yourself and realize your own self-worth, don't worry. You are not alone. Women notoriously are self-sacrificing. In the pages ahead, I will help you re-create yourself from the inside out. In six steps, you will rediscover the new beautiful you.

You have already started to master **Step 1** by buying this book and dreaming of your new transformation. Imagine the changes you want to make. Start by writing down your thoughts about your epiphany when you finish reading this chapter. This will be the first step of your **MAP**—your Makeover Action Plan. Writing down your process will help you to experience it on more of a heartfelt level, and it can serve as a motivational tool as you move along.

In the next chapter, you will begin **Step 2, "Wake Up to Your Dream,"** where you will begin to retrace the steps that brought you to this point in your life and move toward the dream of what you want to become.

Step 3 will focus on **Love, Truth, and Trust—Your Foundations.** These essential chapters will rearrange your thinking and lay the groundwork for **Step 4, "Your Mental Makeover."** This *inside-out* makeover process will ensure your success in changing your appearance, especially full body transformations.

Step 5, "Your Beauty Revealed," will be fun and exciting as you learn how to be more accomplished at makeup, skin care, hairstyling, fitness, and fashion. You will soon possess all the tools that you will need to implement a makeover from head to toe!

Step 6 will actually be planned and written by you . . . more on that later. Even though I am the beauty expert, the most important lesson I can share with you is that only *you* have the power to control your destiny.

From this day forward, remind yourself that you can make decisions to improve your life whether you have experienced your epiphany or just picked up this book out of curiosity. Congratulations! Take a deep breath and pat yourself on the back for acknowledging your personal epiphany and opening the door to caring for yourself. You have taken the first steps along the path to A Beautiful New You. From this day forward, I know that you will enjoy the journey!

Makeover Action Plan: Your Epiphany

Write down your epiphany, the lightbulb moment that indicated to you that you'd had enough. Was it a comment someone made? A photograph of yourself? An experience you had by yourself or with others?

_____

_____

If you feel good about yourself, write down why you bought this book.

_____

_____

What is the single most important change you want to make to yourself physically?

_____

_____

Keep this primary goal in the front of your mind. Remind yourself of this goal often and work toward accomplishing it. Once you've reached that goal, reward yourself. Write down a list of small rewards you will reward yourself with when accomplishing your number one physical goal.

_____

_____

What personal goals would you like to set for yourself that are not ap-pearance related?

    Right now:

_____

_____

    In one month:

_____

_____

    In six months:

_____

_____

    In one year:

_____

_____

    As you progress through this book, refer back to this page from time to time to remind yourself of these goals.

STEP TWO

Wake Up to Your Dream

"When you stop having dreams and ideas—well you can stop altogether."

—MARIAN ANDERSON

2

Beyond the Looking Glass

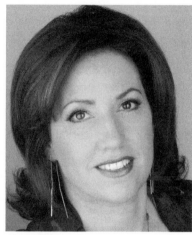

Mary Pierce before

Mary Pierce after

"Once in a while you have to take a break and visit yourself."

—Audrey Giorgi

After twenty-four years of helping women improve their appearances, I still scratch my head trying to figure out why so many of us (myself included) let beauty escape our grasp. It's obvious that women are deeply interested in looking attractive. Look at how we devour fashion magazines, soak up stories about our favorite Hollywood stars, pack the malls week after week, and load up on cosmetics, creams, and concoctions. It appears that women have the desire to look terrific, or at least they start out with the beauty ambition in the early years. Something happens as we progress into our thirties and forties. For me, that something was life. A huge dose of life.

/3 LAURA'S STORY—The Downward Spiral, and Back Up Again

I'll begin by sharing my story. You may see a bit of yourself in it. My tale is no different from the stories of millions of women running through life—working, raising kids, and keeping up (barely) with a crazy schedule. The perpetual motion of my chaotic lifestyle prevented me from taking a moment to really see the negative changes that were happening to me. In my younger years, that wasn't the case. I had my act together when I was a professional model; I was confident, radiant, and loving life.

But at the ripe "old age" of thirty, my modeling career dwindled in Europe, so I returned to the United States and decided to open up my own salon with the manicurist license I had before I became a model. My business grew, and I became more skilled in the beauty industry, obtaining licenses in esthetics, massage, and paramedical makeup. My clientele was thriving, and as my business expanded to two salons, I fell in love and started my family. After the birth of each of my boys, I worked hard to return to my model weight, a feat of which I was very proud (because it took a lot of work).

Just when I thought I had it all, life began to crumble. It was more like an earthquake, really. In a matter of a few months, one of my salons failed, and so did my marriage. Suddenly, I was a single mom without child support faced with caring for two toddlers 24-7 and running a struggling business. Overwhelmed by sorting out the debt created by the salon that closed, and trying to manage the lives of two children, I began to sink into despair and depression. Surviving life one minute at a time became my new routine. I could barely get the children to day care and myself to work on time—the bare minimum was my limit. Meals were prepared by teenagers at the local fast-food restaurants, and I learned to function on four hours of sleep each night. My reality was a blur of endless responsibility. While many moms were deciding in which soccer league to place their little ones, I was trying to keep myself out of bankruptcy and trying to prove to myself that I could be a good mom raising two children alone.

Day in and day out the theme was the same: I lavished my salon clientele with my talents and pampering, and I labored at night to nurture my boys. I focused on working hard to pay off my debts and managed to hold on to the tiny house that I owned. I took care of everything and everybody except *me*. By the time I was forty-three, I had settled into my "life," where fatigue and depression remained my constant companions. My family now tells me that I looked like a frumpy fifty-year-old, although I didn't realize it at the time.

Ironically, as the owner of a full-service salon and day spa, my job was to make women look beautiful and feel wonderful—yet I didn't look or feel great at all. I learned to be proud of the work I did and graciously accepted the raves and compliments from happy clients when they looked at themselves in the mirror. But as I stood behind them while they admired their reflection in the huge mirror before my styling chair, I rarely pulled my focus from the client to myself. As a matter of fact, I had been perfecting the art of ignoring myself for years, convinced that there simply wasn't time to look in a mirror, much less react to what I saw. There certainly wasn't time for makeup or hairstyling, never mind exercising. Other matters were always more urgent and important, like payroll, training new staff, the children's homework, laundry, and bedtime stories.

I was spiraling down deep into "Frumpville," settling into a soft, dumpy figure, sporting an old-fashioned poodle "do" or a freaky, bleached, spiked do, and hoping that wearing glasses would make up for the lack of cosmetics. I never dated, partially because I didn't believe I had the time, so why bother fixing myself up? Another big part of me, however, was purposely pushing attention away from myself, hiding behind the glasses, the dull face, and the lackluster image I'd created. I made a few stabs at changing my looks with hair color or bleach, thinking that I would look hip. I was getting further off the path.

Thankfully, my life changed almost immediately after my "jeans epiphany." That day in front of a dressing room mirror I experienced my "wake-up call" moment. For the first time in seven years, I calculated all of the changes that had taken place; I stared at my own deterioration and let it sink in. That night, I vowed that I would develop a plan to re-create myself.

For the next year, I took one hour each day to implement my plan. I pretended that I was a new client and set out to restyle everything concerning my appearance. Not only did I rely on my own beauty knowledge, I tapped in to the talent and advice of my staff as well. Then, I immersed myself in action—diet, fitness, skin, hair, makeup, clothing, everything! Even though I was always the expert in the salon, I hadn't been giving that expertise to myself. I finally gave myself the permission to use all my skills on me.

Within weeks, even days, people started to notice some changes in my appearance. What happened next was the biggest revelation of my life; their positive remarks fueled me with a powerful drive. My spirits soared, my depression began to dissipate, and a new energy sparked inside of me. *Suddenly I got the daily tasks of running a household and a business done in less time, leaving even more time for me!* I looked forward to going to the gym for a workout and cheerfully set the alarm clock a little earlier so that I could put on my makeup. I discarded my out-of-date, thick glasses and invested in a supply of disposable contact lenses. As I continued to enjoy what I saw in the mirror, I was happy and, for the first time in seven years, felt alive!

It was a year after my comeback that I slowly started to figure out that what happened to me was happening to women everywhere. Life has sucked the spirit of beauty right out of us, even the desire. For me, it happened slowly over seven dreary years of putting myself last. Your setback may have been more sudden. I didn't like what I saw one day when I looked in the mirror. I had to change. If you can "mirror" this experience, then it may be time for you to change also. To do that I am going to put a big bold mirror up in front of you and encourage you to take a really good look. Then we're going to examine ourselves even more deeply, beyond the looking glass, for some answers that will guide you through your transformation.

To See or Not to See?

That is the question. In the last year, how many of you have really *looked* at yourself in the mirror? Did you absorb what you saw? I didn't for years and years and get this . . . I was a beauty expert *and* worked all day in front of a huge mirror! I became an expert at seeing my outline in the mirror but not really observing what I looked like. Does this sound a bit like you? What we are doing when we look but don't see is avoiding what we don't *want* to see. We choose not to see elements about our appearance that we don't approve of. We learn to tune ourselves out, a technique I call "blurring out" the image in the mirror.

⅓ MARY'S STORY

Mary Pierce and I met each other at our sons' school. Our shared experience was to devote ourselves completely to our children, attending field trips and classroom parties and dutifully steering homework and progress. This mother of two boys also accepted the heavy responsibility of caring for her own mother who has Alzheimer's. Mary learned quickly to bypass mirrors. "I was so overwhelmed I felt like a victim. My health was slipping. I was very anxious and not sleeping well. Thinking about how I looked was the farthest thing down the list. Laura gave me the key to my life."

Mary's downward spiral began when an on-the-job injury left her with neck and shoulder pain. Feeling defeated, she stopped exercising, gained weight, and started blurring out her image in the mirror. Depression crept in as she believed she would never get back into exercise and regain her strong and slender body.

Courageously, Mary returned to the gym after observing my transformation. She approached me at school events with curiosity about my weight-lifting routine. Mary was frustrated with a lack of results struggling with her traditional aerobic workout. I shared my exercise routine and techniques with her (which are detailed in chapter 16), and within two months of committed work, Mary had lost seventeen pounds! She also has gained the strength she needed in her supporting muscles to relieve a lot of the pain she had from her injury—without reinjuring herself in the process. She says that her chiropractor is amazed at her progress and mobility. Mary told me with pride she is now physically and emotionally stronger. "I feel so much more sure of myself. I feel like I can achieve anything. My life is back in perspective. I'm much calmer and more patient."

The bonus for Mary is that she has so much more confidence. As her health dwindled, Mary helplessly had watched as every last remnant of her self-esteem disappeared. Now Mary feels that she can be present without feeling like wallpaper in the background. And she should! "I won't give up on a problem now. And if I can't solve the problem, I don't feel guilty and like a failure."

Exercise is therapy for Mary. "I am no longer just a task-performing machine called Mom. I have allowed myself to have a personality again, and I'm giving myself permission to have my own hobbies and spend time doing totally frivolous things that I would have never done before. Surprise-surprise, my family is enjoying me more too."

One son now calls her "Slim," and her husband sings her praises to others about her accomplishments. She told me she has more energy for all the people in her life who need her. "I am a much better daughter and mother. My husband and children are treating me with more respect. They realize I have a life now and I am an equal partner. I no longer say I *need* time for myself, I *take* time for myself. I assumed spending time at the gym would be at the cost of someone else (my kids, my mom, my job, etc.). What I have realized since dedicating myself to getting healthy is that not only has this not taken anything away from my family, but it has enhanced the quality of all my relationships."

By avoiding the pain of our real image in the mirror, we can continue on with life just the way it is, feeling sorry for ourselves and feeling like there is no way out. We deny what is in front of us so we don't have to change. Denial is the greatest beauty sin, and the first obstacle you must face to recapture your beauty.

What causes denial if every woman wants to be beautiful? Ask any woman; she'll give you a list of reasons or excuses all centered around a common theme of self-worthiness. See if these denials sound familiar:

- I don't have time to look in the mirror.
- My husband loves me no matter what I look like.
- My children don't care if I'm a little overweight.
- I'm too busy to fix myself up.
- Now that I'm home with the baby, nobody sees me.
- Everybody gains a little weight as they get older.
- I'm not nineteen anymore.
- I look okay for thirty, forty, fifty.
- I can't afford to go to a salon.
- I've never been the high-maintenance type.

Sticking by these stories will definitely keep you in the "blur" when you catch a glimpse of yourself in the mirror. Being in denial is a secure position. You don't have to change. Life goes on.

The preceding denials are the same words I have heard over and over from my clients. I have learned to read between the lines and hold the client's hand to force them to look beyond the looking glass at what I believe they truly want, to live their lives and be gorgeous at the same time.

I recently met a client named Diana who was denying what she really wanted, which was to feel better about herself. Although she lived two hours away managing a small farm, she justified a quick trip to town to see me hoping I could make her glamorous by way of a low-maintenance haircut. "Low maintenance?" I asked. "Why?"

"Because I run a busy farm and nobody sees me!" I paused for a moment to draw her full attention and gently asked, "Don't you have any mirrors on that farm?" Her eyes crinkled up as she chuckled, immediately getting the jest of my jab. "You're right, I don't want low maintenance. I want fabulous!" Good for you, Diana.

Stop denying what you see in the mirror that needs attention. Stop denying yourself the right to be beautiful.

20-20 Vision

Improve your eyesight. Have the courage to take in and digest what you see in the mirror. Not everyone will have the same issues or reality. I imagine for most of you, the hardest element to face will be the size and/or shape of your body. Women have been fixated on their bodies forever. Don't feel alone if you are slightly or largely overweight—most of America is. If your body pleases you but you haven't changed your hair since high school, don't be afraid to acknowledge that. Your hair is one of the easiest features to change right away. Take a look at your skin. Does it reveal your age (or worse, make you look older than you actually are) or do you have everybody guessing? Whatever you see that pleases or displeases you, acknowledge it. Write down your observations. Simply by improving your eyesight and focusing on your real image you have taken the first step in responsibility. When denial gives way to responsibility, change can take place.

Beauty Shame

For three days after my epiphany I walked around with my head down muttering to myself, "What have I done? How could I do this to my body?" The shock and panic I felt turned into shame. I had been a high achiever, a model, a beauty expert! Was I nuts? No, but I sure felt like a hypocrite. I also felt the black cloud of thinking that this was as good as it would get. I could never get my beautiful figure and image back. You may benefit someday in the future by reminding yourself of how far you spiraled down, but for now, try to channel the feeling of shame toward something positive. Feeling the shame temporarily is good, for it means that you value yourself after all. Examine the power of the negative emotion and let it fuel you with energy to recommit to yourself.

Forgiveness

When you look in the mirror and take it all in, learn to forgive yourself. The reasons why you shelved yourself for a while probably felt honorable at the time. Most women are creatures of caring. Our genetic "defect" that comes with the loving nature is that we tend to love others more than ourselves. Forgiving yourself, then caring for yourself, will be the next steps toward change.

Perfect Vision to Dream Your Dream

What I want you to really think about is what you would want the mirror to reflect if you could wave a magic wand. If you could, would you like to be gorgeous? A knockout? A head turner? Be honest, of course you would. No matter what a woman tells me in her modesty or with humility, I never believe that she prefers to be dowdy, old-fashioned, frumpy, plain, or even simple. I want you to live your dream, fulfill your perfect vision of what you want to feel when you walk into a room. What you visualize, you can make happen.

Through the Looking Glass and Back

Never be afraid to look back down the road that led you to your epiphany and the long look in the mirror. By retracing the steps we took down that road, we can discover the pathway back to beauty.

Whatever was going on in your life that gobbled up your radiance and glamour must be put in balance. Change things around. Reverse your thinking and take a new direction. Your "about-face" will put you back on track. The answer in how to move forward lies deep in the mirror, beyond the looking glass. I will help guide you through it.

Remember the story of Alice in Wonderland? Alice fell into the looking glass and went on a big adventure. That is what I wish for you. I can tell you from my own personal transformation experience that it is never too late to change the way you look. I did it well into my forties. You get to start over, and I believe you will love the adventure. All along the way you will be shadowed lovingly by your new self, the one who cares about you.

Makeover Action Plan: Beyond the Looking Glass

LOOKING GLASS SELF-EVALUATION

Which of your physical attributes do you like most? (i.e., your beautiful hair, blue eyes, etc.)_____

_____

What physical attributes would you like to change?_____

_____

_____

Was there a time in your life when you really liked the way you looked and felt? That's your starting point. Write about it.

_____

_____

Now write about what happened in your life that took away your radiance._____

_____

_____

Once you trace your path backward to recognize what circumstances led you down the path away from your radiance and beauty, you can begin to re-create your circumstances and take a new path to beauty.

Do you look in the mirror and quickly look away in disgust or shame? The first step to becoming friends with the mirror is to *look* and *see*. The next step is to know you are human and forgive yourself.

Write down what makes you shameful when you look in the mirror._____

_____

Now, change the feelings of shame to a commitment toward change. For example: I am ashamed of how much weight I have gained. Pledge: I will begin today eating healthy foods and make it a goal to reduce my weight to a healthy level.

Name one or two ways you can take better care of yourself starting now. These can be "baby steps," like making sure you drink enough water each day, making a doctor's appointment you've been putting off, or going to bed earlier.

_____

_____

PERFECT VISION

The first step in realizing your dream is to visualize it. It's no different from an Olympic gymnast who visualizes every move in a balance beam routine before performing. What you wish for or visualize, you can accomplish. You can make your dreams come true.

In one sentence, describe the way you would like to look if you could wave a magic wand. Remember, the goal is to make realistic goals that you can achieve on your own without plastic surgery!

_____

_____

3

The Power of Beauty

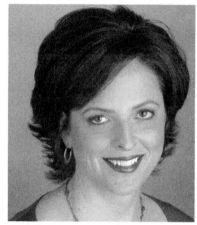

Barbara Arrowsmith before

Barbara Arrowsmith after

"I don't want life to imitate art. I want life to be art."

—Carrie Fisher

"Hey Mom," called my youngest son, Johnny, as he walked into the bathroom while I was fixing my hair. He was ten at the time and it was exactly a year since my epiphany, and I had just lost over seventy pounds. "Does being overweight make you grouchy?" My puzzled expression caused him to elaborate. "I mean, when you were bigger, you were always grouchy and sad. Now you seem happy all the time. I was just wondering if being chubby makes people grumpy."

At that moment, I realized what an unhappy person I had become during those years of neglecting myself. Even a ten-year-old could sense the difference in my persona. Self-neglect created a change in my personality, my self-esteem, and my outlook on life. Restoring a healthy body and radiant image did the opposite. My self-esteem soared, and my negative disposition melted away. I loved life again and enthusiastically charged ahead with working, raising children, and tackling projects. The difference in my outlook was like night and day, all because I started to take an interest in myself again. *That is the power of beauty.*

Beauty is difficult to define, yet we know it when we see it. Since antiquity we have been infatuated with beauty, yet it remains somewhat of a mystery. In ancient times, tattoos, rings through ears and noses, body painting, and other customs were employed to enhance beauty. In other cultures across the globe, today's standards of beauty vary immensely from the Western ideals depicted in glossy fashion magazines. In the twenty-first century, we still see tattoos and piercing, but now we've added hair dyeing, waxing, Botox, and so on. All of these sophisticated methods are solely for improving appearance and creating beauty.

But why? As a witness to thousands of makeovers, I have seen how an improved appearance can improve self-image for woman after woman. Studies have shown that an attractive individual appears to have a better chance at social and career success, but my purpose here is personal, not business. I want to help you reach new emotional heights as you discover your own beauty. It does not matter if you are pretty or plain, your beauty is a constant—as much a part of you as your brain—and therefore it is important for your personal growth.

BARBARA'S STORY

Barbara Arrowsmith always believed it's the beauty inside a person that counts. She shared that message with class after class of adolescents in her career as a middle school teacher. Barbara admits she embraced that philosophy so much that she didn't make much of an effort in her own everyday appearance. But there was another reason she resisted. "My hair had a personality of its own. Thick, coarse, and curly. I'd wake up every day never knowing what it was going to look like. In fog and rain my hair expands." It was too much work to make her hair look good every day. She sought help from hairstylist after hairstylist. Fifteen salons later she still didn't have the answer. Her sister suggested Barbara visit my salon. I invited Barbara to be a "Monday Makeover" on my weekly appearance on a local TV newscast on KXTV in Sacramento. After a cut and color and application with Mane Tame, a salon product, and a hot iron treatment, Barbara was gorgeous and happy. When her before and after pictures appeared side by side on the screen, there was an audible gasp from those in the studio. "At that moment I began to feel different. I began to feel my best," Barbara told me later.

After her Monday Makeover, Barbara learned that if she spent just a little extra time each day on herself, she could turn heads. "My students stopped dead in their tracks as they passed me in the hall. Some said they didn't recognize me and wondered who the new teacher was." Her confidence soared and she opened her mind to the possibility that outer beauty was important, too. "I didn't expect the emotional lift I experienced after paying attention to my outward self. I am much more approachable to other people now. One parent commented to me, 'You look younger now than when you taught my son eight years ago.' "

Barbara hasn't wavered from her mission to get students to see beauty from within. The forty-five-year-old teacher deals daily with adolescents with prickly personalities who experiment with purple hair and black makeup. Now Barbara has her own personal experiment to share with them. "In some way I have outgrown my own adolescence some thirty years late. I have come to see that now the beauty within me has a more direct pathway to my students and to others."

Over the course of the year after her makeover Barbara even dropped a dress size. I am especially grateful to see Barbara walk in my salon because I know she just drove two hours from her home in Santa Rosa. A four-hour round-trip! She made my day when she told me that the results of her makeover were worth every mile.

Barbara learned that her appearance positively influenced everyone around her. Our appearance is more than a façade—it communicates to others how we feel about ourselves. A well-groomed appearance indicates pride and self-esteem, among other things. It may not be fair, but most of us judge others to some extent on how they look. The manner in which a person dresses can communicate wealth, social status, organization, business status, and so on. Your body shape, hair, and makeup (or the lack of makeup) can also send signals to others, negative and positive. The most important factor you will communicate to others when it comes to your appearance is the way you feel about yourself. Think about that. *Your self-esteem will be communicated by the way you look.*

Not so, you say? Let's take a quick look at some other examples of beauty affecting the way we think.

It's a Beautiful Life

People by nature are lovers of beauty. We see beauty in nature all around us. Snow-capped mountains. A meadow of bright yellow daffodils. The Grand Canyon. Beauty amazes us, delights and thrills us. We are impressed by beautiful things that represent achievement and effort. The Grand Canyon is a marvel of beauty, awe, and wonder because it took millions of years to create. We hold the same reverence for beautiful works of art. The appreciation you may feel for the statue of David carved from stone by Michelangelo is largely due to how difficult it was to accomplish. Art is one of the strongest examples of beauty I can think of that exists purely for our enjoyment and admiration. Could we live without art? Of course we could. But why would you want to?

We could also live without parks. Can you imagine your town or city without the beauty of Mother Nature? We are a society that plans for and includes beauty in our lives. City planners include art, interesting architecture, and parks when designing a city. Nobody wants to live in a town that is designed purely for function, including only streets, sidewalks, and buildings.

In your own neighborhood, beauty is displayed and interpreted. Think about your impression of a homeowner with a beautifully manicured lawn and excellent landscaping. The effort the homeowner makes shows a sense of pride. Whether you want to admit it or not, you will decide that this homeowner is probably more intelligent and successful than the neighbor across the street with the overgrown lawn and a house with peeling paint.

The absolute same conclusions will be made when it comes to your personal appearance. Does your exterior show others that you take pride in yourself? Or does it look like the homeowner is on vacation? One of the reasons that people notice the way we look is because it demonstrates a level of effort and accomplishment. It's not easy to be fit and well groomed. It requires time, attention, and effort.

I love to tell the story of a client named Helen. For two years she would come to see me for a supershort, low-maintenance cut. I thought the cropped do made her look masculine and so I slowly tried to sneak in the suggestion to grow it out. "Nope!" Helen would say. "I don't have time to style it." I knew that Helen was retired, so I finally asked what she did with her time. As it turns out, Helen is an avid gardener and spends all of her time every day in her award-winning garden. It was evident that those plants and shrubs gave her a sense of pride and satisfaction. Still, I believed that, deep down, Helen had that same pride in her own appearance; she just needed a little help seeing the connection between pride and her own outer beauty. On her fifth visit to my salon, I gently repeated my suggestion that she let me give her a more flattering hairstyle. She sighed and declared once again, "I don't have a lot of time to mess with myself. My garden takes up all of my time." I replied, as I looked directly into her blue eyes, "But Helen, you can't take your garden around with you!" She got it immediately. I could see the lightbulb turn on in her head. "You're right, Laura . . . go ahead." Helen still has a beautiful garden, but she also looks fantastic while she's working in it!

Pride Versus Whatever

For many of us, it may feel as if the last several years have been the "whatever" years. "Why should I fix my hair?" "Who cares if I get fat?" "What does it matter if I wear makeup or not?" We are a society that has embraced the word *whatever,* when it comes to just about everything. In my family, I have banned this word and gotten back to having a sense of pride in everything we do. My boys have developed a sense of pride also in their daily responsibilities. They brush their teeth more thoroughly, comb their hair, attack their homework, clean their rooms, and help with chores. *No more whatever.* This policy began when I started taking pride in myself again. Pride is infectious. If you show it in yourself, it will spread to others in your family. Take "whatever" out of your vocabulary (and your family's) today!

Exponential Beauty Power

Over the years of making thousands of women over I've witnessed a phenomenon I call exponential beauty power. It's the increased energy women experience from taking care of themselves. This surge of energy is created when a woman realizes her own importance and the value of looking and feeling like a million bucks.

When you have pride in yourself and look your best, others will notice, but most important, you will be empowered to accomplish more with a greater amount of vitality and satisfaction. You will demonstrate your self-worth to others as well as yourself. This is the power of beauty I am talking about.

My heart leaps with joy when I help clients experience the power of *their* beauty. If you have never witnessed what I am talking about, you soon will and your life will never be the same. If you have experienced the "power," perhaps you lost it because you forgot how much it improved your life. The simple but incredible fact is that you can harness the power anytime that you want, once you make the decision to reclaim your radiance. Here are some exercises to help you tap in to the power of beauty, inside and out. That's the beauty of beauty!

Makeover Action Plan: Your Beauty Power

BE AN OBSERVER OF BEAUTY TODAY

Connect with and notice beauty every day. If someone looks pleasing to you, compliment that person on his or her appearance. Appreciate nature's unfoldings every day. Enjoy works of art. By connecting with beauty you will naturally radiate beauty from yourself. Create beauty with a simple crafts project you enjoy. Redecorate a small part of your home. Plant flowers. Paint or draw with a child. Write a poem or a note about the power of beauty in your journal.

Remember the last time someone complimented you on your appearance? Write about that now. What, in particular, were you complimented on? Your hair, clothing, or overall look?

_____

_____

_____

That's the power of beauty. How did the compliment make you feel?

START YOUR LOOK BOOK

Get a simple manila folder and a couple of fashion magazines. Cruise through the magazines and tear out the photographs of models whose look you admire. This folder will become more important later. For now, just collect faces that appeal to you. By looking at what appeals to you, you will begin to form your "dream look." Keep the folder handy, for example, on the dresser in your bedroom or on the kitchen counter, and add to it regularly. You will use your look book extensively in the chapters ahead.

4

Imagine the All New You

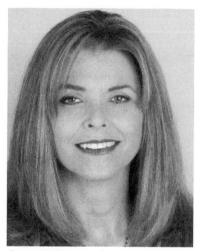

Susan McFerson before

Susan McFerson after

"Imagination is the highest kite that can fly."

—LAUREN BACALL

Judy arrived at my salon ten minutes early, my first client of the day. As I looked up from my appointment book, I could see a little excitement mixed in with her obvious nervousness. Trying out a new hairstylist seems to be a stressful event for many people. Judy was earmarked in my schedule as a "new request" client referred by watching the Monday Makeover segment on television. As we shook hands, I looked directly into her eyes, trying to assess her level of confidence and self-esteem. Her smile was sincere, but I sensed that she was unsure of herself. I found her face to be fresh, natural, and pretty, but her features were concealed by a heavy wall of bangs and overpowered by thick shoulder-length hair. Her eyes were a pale gray-blue, framed by mousy brown hair that was graying at the roots. Her facial features were beautifully balanced, but she was thirty to forty pounds overweight, making her face a little full. Judy was probably in her late thirties but appeared closer to fifty. My creative excitement began to stir. I couldn't wait to show Judy how a makeover would change her image and lift her spirits.

While Judy settled in my chair, I situated myself with my back to the mirror, facing her. I like to communicate with a client face-to-face and watch how they interact with their image in the mirror. Seeing their reaction to their own reflection is one of the ways I get to grasp their self-image.

"So, Judy, what brings you here to my chair?"

"I saw your makeovers on television and thought you could make me over starting with my hair." Most of the women I consult with come to me for a new hairstyle or design and consider this the most important step in a makeover. What I ask next usually surprises and puzzles the client: "Before I consider a hairstyle for you, let's talk about a bigger picture. What is the image you want to present? How do you want to look?"

Judy's brows drew together slightly, reflecting her caution with the tone of her voice: "I thought you would tell me what style would be right for me; you know, the best style for my face."

I smiled and nodded my head. "You could wear a lot of different styles because you have a beautiful face and an excellent head of thick hair. I could pick a current style for you that would compliment your features, but I don't want a cookie cutter version of you based on a styling book. I want to give you the look you've always dreamed of. I want to make you look and feel beautiful."

Judy's reply is the number one response I hear daily as a beauty expert. "I don't know about the beautiful part, but I want a new style that I can do in five minutes." Again I try to redirect Judy back to her dream. "If I could wave a magic wand and create any look you want, what would that look be? Glamorous and sexy? Fresh and natural? Sophisticated and professional? Or all of the above?"

I paused and watched Judy's face. She turned to her own image in the mirror and squirmed a bit. Shrugging her shoulders, she said, "I really don't know. I haven't thought about it much; I'm just a busy mom and want a change."

Judy's consultation and responses to my prodding are not uncommon. Her experience prior to our meeting was to go to the salon when she felt in a rut. Her basic beauty needs were pretty much limited to a new haircut, putting a home color rinse on her roots when she couldn't stand the gray anymore, and splurging on a few new makeup items a couple of times a year. *She was steering her own boat without really knowing where she wanted to go.* My goal was to get her to commit to a destination, the image she dreamed of having. Together we would then devise a plan to achieve her goal.

That day, I gave Judy a slight revision of her haircut and taught her how to style it in ten minutes. We agreed to forgo a major haircut change until she had time to design her new look. Before she left, I gave Judy a homework assignment. I asked that she look for photographs from her lifetime when she felt good about herself and loved the way she looked. She agreed to come back in four weeks for hair color and a makeup lesson, and she promised to bring her scrapbook.

Many women defer to me and other stylists as the beauty experts who should decide their new look for them. I appreciate their compliment but always, always, always bring them in on the decision-making process. It's not unlike how an interior designer evaluates your tastes, desire, and even budget when fashioning the rooms in your house. Would it feel comfortable to walk into your home that a designer made over without any direction or input from you? Of course not. The way I see it, you have to live with your appearance just as you have to live with the design of your home. Beauty advice should be married with your tastes, likes and dislikes, and especially your lifestyle. If you haven't been a "makeup" person, you won't be comfortable applying a bagful of cosmetics every day.

✍ SUSAN'S STORY

When she was a little girl, Susan McFerson wanted to be like her mother, who was a dancer. At age five, Susan began dance lessons. Ballet and jazz classes and performances continued through high school. In college, she choreographed dance programs and traveled the world as part of the singing group Up With People. As a blond, gorgeous, and shapely entertainer Susan knew the importance of staying physically fit and always looking her best. Until menopause. "I went from the prom queen era to the menopause era and it rocked my boat."

Going through her forties made Susan rethink her regimen for staying attractive and taking care of her body. Society was telling her that a woman pushing fifty shouldn't be sexy and slender with long hair. "I kept asking myself what camp was I in? Should I grow old and keep quiet or keep working to look the way I want to look?" The married mother of two girls, ages six and fourteen, said she wanted to be respectable, and in the process she relented to the pressure of low expectations. Susan gained thirty pounds and wore her greasy hair pulled back. It was an appearance that forced her to hide behind a telephone pole one day when she saw an old friend she hadn't seen in twenty years walk through a parking lot. "Later I thought, if that is my reaction, I don't want to be that way. I'm not comfortable."

Susan was too stubborn to give up. Her need to celebrate her femininity was affirmed by me as she visited my salon for hair services. I did not cut her hair short! Her long, light brown hair with gold highlights is stunning. A sixty-year-old woman who is a stranger went out of her way to compliment Susan, who was shopping in a clothing store. "You have a beautiful head of hair and I'm glad there are fifty-year-old women out there who have the courage to look sexy," the stranger said. The woman gave Susan a high five and defiantly said, "I'm not cutting my long hair!" Susan said, "Neither am I!"

You have to work harder on your appearance in your forties and fifties, but Susan says it is worth it. Her husband appreciates her beauty, and Susan feels confident about facing any challenge in life. She encouraged her younger sister, Barbara Arrowsmith, to visit my salon. (You just read about Barbara in chapter 3, "The Power of Beauty.")

Susan's energy and passion for dance has continued from age five to fifty. She is now taking tap lessons so she can join an over-fifty tap troupe. "I can't sit still when I hear jazz. The music infuses me with energy and gives me hope for a better tomorrow."

Susan suggests that women in the forties and fifties should embrace where they are and never give up. As for herself she says, "I'm going to have lip gloss on when I take my last breath, and it will probably be hot pink."

Follow Your Instincts, Follow Your Dream

Think back to your first day of kindergarten, the first day of school. You probably went off to school in a new dress with your hair neatly tied in pretty ribbons. Going to school was a big event, and making a good impression was important. The desire to look our best continues and even grows through the high school and college years. For some, the sense of pride or the need to make a good impression lasts forever. The point of this chapter is to spark your thinking about what it is you really want when it comes to presenting yourself to the world and, most important, to the mirror. If you started out in your youth looking "together" and enjoying making a favorable impression, I want you to realize that those actions were admirable. Common sense and basic social instinct drove you to make the effort to look nice every day. If you've lost that drive or are inconsistent in presenting the image you really want to have, then go back and tap in to your instincts and follow your dream. Go for the "you" that you really want to be, from head to toe.

⌁ LISA'S STORY

Lisa Wibberly developed that fantasy about the way she wanted to look and worked hard to make it came true beginning when she was a little girl. Growing up in Woodland, California, Lisa noticed that some of her relatives were overweight. She was concerned that family influences would lead her to an unhealthy lifestyle. Entering junior high school, Lisa felt peer pressure to look good. She loved snow and water skiing, but also took up running and aerobics classes as a young girl. As an independent-thinking young woman she vowed she would always take care of herself. "It has to do with self-respect and the rewards from self-respect are great. Staying in shape increases my self-esteem and makes me a better person all the way around," she told me.

As a mother her motivation goes beyond her own physical benefits. "I want to be an example for the boys." Lisa's three boys are learning by example and word about the importance of good nutrition and exercise. "My sons respect themselves more now because they know that soda, candy, and junk food are extremely rare treats in our home." This busy mom holds down a full-time job as a youth leader at church but religiously exercises every week. She is faithful to running three to five miles five days a week and she attends a Pilates class three times a week. The youngsters in her youth group are getting it too. "I tell them that God has given them a gift in their body. What I do with it is my choice. I choose to take care of myself in a way that makes me feel good."

One day during a visit to my salon, I discovered another motive for Lisa's healthy philosophy. I overheard her tell another client, "I believe it's important to look good for my husband. He deserves it." I stopped what I was doing and said, "Lisa, forgive me for eavesdropping, but what did you say?" She elaborated, "You get what you give in a relationship. It's an honor to take care of myself for him." Lisa's husband appreciates her commitment and dedication to a healthy lifestyle and it has inspired him to stay in shape and eat better. "It's nice to know my husband takes pride in himself for me."

Lisa Wibberly is realizing the extra benefits of staying in shape and taking care of her appearance: increased confidence, more joy, and a great relationship with her husband and sons. Good for her!

Your Own Exterior Designer

What's the look *you* love? What is your dream look? For some of you, zeroing in on your ideal look will be easy. Perhaps you want to look like you did at another time in your life. The prom? Your wedding day? At your five-year class reunion? How did you feel at that time? Radiant and confident? Others may have the experience that they have never felt outwardly attractive or appealing. Perhaps you were attractive but lived in the shadow of a prettier mother or sister. Your perception was that your looks didn't measure up. Whatever the case, you can design your transformation based on your joyful past or by your imagination. The important point is that your transformation begins in your creative mind. I believe the secret formula to any successful accomplishment requires three simple steps. Think it. Believe it. Do it. For now, let's address the "think it" step—the imagination stage.

What do you want to look like? What image would you like to project? I ask this question a lot in my salon chair, especially when I have a new client who wants me to make them over. I believe that the best answer lies within the heart of the woman I am counseling. You must search your own heart for the answer that will best serve you. Do you want to look sexy and glamorous? Yes, of course you would; who wouldn't? How about looking sophisticated? Mysterious and exotic? I want you to really think and explore your heart and your imagination without trying to talk yourself out of anything. Your dream can be achieved; you simply have to start with a dream. There is a neat exercise coming up to get you started on your new look.

Once you have imagined your new look you need to believe that you can achieve that which you've dreamed about. The next section of this book will guide you through the very important process of believing in yourself. After you become a believer you will be ready for the "do it" part. That will come later in this book and is the most fun part. For now, let's continue on with the creating and planning of your new image.

Picture This

All professional models have a portfolio or a "look book," a collection of photographs representing what they can look like. Some models have a very stylized image that doesn't vary too much, but most can pull off dozens of looks expressing different emotions and attitudes. Before I had the experience of modeling and developing a portfolio, I thought there was only one way of appearing. Day in and day out, one would always look the same, except for gaining a few pounds or aging. My ten years posing in front of the camera allowed me to see myself in many different ways. Trust me when I tell you that with the right makeup and hair techniques, desire, and attitude, you too could have an entire portfolio of looks as well. Think of yourself as a model or actress, able to jump into any persona you were hired to do. Don't limit yourself to the image you have had, especially if you aren't happy with it. It's time to try something different, fresh, and exciting.

Creating Your Look Book

I want you to make a portfolio or a look book for yourself to help you communicate your new image and design to yourself and your beauty professionals. It doesn't have to be fancy. A simple binder will do. The first step is to put the magazine tearout sheets you collected in the chapter 3 MAP activity into your binder. If you haven't started this project yet, don't fret; start today by cruising through magazines and catalogs, cutting out pictures of beautiful women who attract your attention. Organize the pictures in designated sections including:

1. The Total Look
2. Hairstyles
3. Makeup
4. Clothing

By collecting photos of women and styles you love, you will stay focused on the exterior design you'd love for yourself. Never talk yourself out of trying to achieve for yourself the beauty and glamour you admire that other women project. If they can . . . *you can.*

Keep your look book with you all the time or at least in your car or desk. It will be your guide for every beauty appointment or for shopping trips. You can continually update it, and of course you should. Part of taking care of yourself is staying current and keeping up with fresh ideas. Make a commitment to get out of the rut and into the groove, but resist the temptation to become a fashion slave. How? Use your common sense first of all. Sprinkle in the latest trend along with classics. Up ahead in chapter 14, "The Cure for Your Closet," I will share my secret for freshening up your wardrobe. For now, let your magazine tearouts in your look book inspire you.

Putting Your Plan into Action

Once you have an image design, start taking action. You don't have to wait for someone else to help you. You can start with small steps like imitating some of the makeup or hairstyles you see in your look book. I promise that in the pages ahead, you will receive positive reinforcement to make your dream come true along with technical support you can learn on your own or with the help of your salon professionals. Now that you have a visual plan for yourself to view and to help convey your desire to others, you can move forward with your transformation. Last, never forget that you designed the plan and therefore it is the right look for you. It is your dream.

Makeover Action Plan: Use Your Imagination

Here's a fun exercise to get you thinking about what you really want to look like instead of being stuck in a rut. Circle the answers and fill in the blanks.

1. I like to feel sexy and glamorous
   a. all the time.
   b. only when I go out on dates or special occasions.
   c. only in a private, romantic situation.
   d. never.

2. Circle the words that best describe the image you want to project (you may circle as many as you'd like).

glamorous	beautiful	professional
sexy	sophisticated	conservative
exotic	natural	mature
young	radiant	mysterious
wild	trendy	cute

3. Name one friend or family member whose appearance you find very attractive or appealing._____

   _____

4. Using the list from number 2, write the words that describe her.

   _____

   _____

5. Name three celebrities who you think represent the epitome of beauty.

    a._____

    b._____

    c._____

After filling in all the blanks, you should start to see a trend in the way you view what you find attractive in a woman and what you want others to see when you walk in a room. If you are honest with yourself, you probably want to turn heads and be admired. If given a choice, very few women want to disappear or seem invisible. This exercise should give you a clearer view of what your desire is deep down. Don't chase that desire away!

Write about your dream look—what do you want to look like? Be specific from head to toe!_____

_____

_____

_____

Reminder. Start or add to your look book if you haven't already. Having visual images from magazines and catalogs will help you focus on what your dream look is and will help you communicate with hairstylists, salesclerks, and so on.

Love, Truth, and Trust—
Your Foundations

"The very least you do in your life is to figure out what you hope for. And the most you can do is to live inside that hope."

—BARBARA KINGSOLVER

5

Giving Yourself Permission

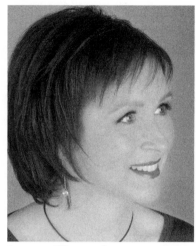

Lynnette Weaver before

Lynnette Weaver after

"Desire. Ask. Believe. Receive."

—STELLA TERRILL MANN

You just received an invitation to a formal evening wedding. One of your best friends is getting married, and everyone you know from high school will be there. What's the first thing that you think? What you will wear, right? You daydream about making an extra effort so you will look fabulous. Perhaps you will go all out and get your hair and makeup done professionally at a salon.

You'll jump through hoops to look good for a big job interview. Remember how long it used to take you to get ready for a big date? These special circumstances motivate women to take action to look beautiful. Why? Why do we need a special reason or permission to fix ourselves up?

I believe the answer is because people are motivated when they want to make a positive impression on others. Impressing others was modeled for us all of our lives. Remember the first day of school, dressing up for Sunday school, and how important it was to look fabulous the first time you met your mate's parents? After we've made this first impression, the desire to keep up appearances can fade or evaporate. Once we feel accepted, we grow comfortable and lose some of the desire to impress.

When we're alone, we think "Why bother?" There is no one to impress except ourselves. What does that say about our self-worth if we make an effort solely for others? Aren't you important to yourself? Absolutely you are. Clearly, you know how significant you are to your family, friends, and coworkers. Now you need to make the connection in your mind that you recognize your value. Acknowledge it. Embrace your worth. Then give yourself permission. Permission for what? To care for yourself. You permit yourself to be a worker, a student, or a caretaker. Why is it so difficult to provide for your own personal and emotional needs? The answer lies in the very nature of women.

Nurturers or Martyrs?

Women have a natural ability to nurture, comfort, soothe, and care for others. It comes by instinct because we are designed to bear and raise children. Even without having children, many females find a way to express their innate maternal instincts. It doesn't matter whether we are between relationships, have a boyfriend, or are married with children—we cook and clean, massage, fuss, dote, fix, heal, and sometimes smother those we love. We offer patience, attention, affection, and compassion because it satisfies our natural desire to be caretakers. Caring for others gives us a sense of pride, makes us feel needed and vital. The vitality can be addictive. It energizes us. But that energy can fizzle. Giving to everyone around you can leave your fuel tank empty. A time will come when you have to fill up. To fill up you must take a break from giving up all of yourself for others. You must refill yourself by taking care of *you*.

LYNNETTE'S STORY

Lynnette Weaver was very young when she got married the first time—unfortunately the marriage deteriorated a few years later. In her thirties, she met the man of her dreams and married a second time. She remembers being so in love that she felt like a princess. She always had great-looking hair and loved wearing makeup to please herself and her new husband.

They wanted children, so at thirty-eight, Lynnette underwent fertility treatment and found herself expecting three babies instead of one. And here is where her story of beauty deterioration begins. She was restricted to modified bed rest, spending hours in the recliner, watching television. Her personal appearance was the first thing to go. "There were points in the pregnancy that taking a shower required immense effort, let alone fixing myself up!"

The babies were born ten weeks early, and all three had to stay in the hospital initially. Their arrival home was staggered between October and December, the last baby entering the house on Christmas Eve. During those months Lynnette's life was a whirlwind, darting back and forth to the hospital and trying to care for the babies. To make matters worse, her strong, glossy hair—one benefit of pregnancy—began falling out in huge clumps! "My personal 'get-ready routine' consisted of showering and pulling back my thinning hair in a ponytail." When little Robert, Byron, and Chad were finally all together at home, Lynnette was housebound for the first three months. Between caring for the babies (including pumping milk—so very unglamorous!) and keeping the house up, she was so fatigued that she couldn't carry on a conversation.

Prior to the birth, Lynnette had always worked in a professional office and cared about the way she looked; she'd worn makeup and fixed her hair. Once she became homebound, she settled for wearing athletic pants and T-shirts; huge clumps of hair continued fleeing from her scalp. "I was discouraged to say the least. I felt unattractive and depressed. Caring for myself just didn't seem like a priority anymore."

Being home every day, she saw my makeover segments on television. "I knew that's what I needed even though I never could justify spending the money on myself. I guess a makeover seemed frivolous. It didn't seem like a *need* at the time—like home improvements or something like that." But she religiously watched the show for several weeks and was just amazed at the transformation of the people. Finally, she called my salon and was chosen for a television makeover. Her makeover was amazing!

Lynnette's epiphany came when, at the end of her new motherhood rope, she realized she had nothing to lose and a whole lot to regain.

"All of a sudden my personal beauty routine is an important *need* and not a frivolity. Keeping myself up makes me feel good about myself and energized to care for my lovely triplets!"

After the makeover, a friend of Lynnette remarked, "Wow, you look great!" Another person said, "I knew there was a pretty woman in there somewhere!" At that moment, Lynnette thought, "Okay, people really do notice how you look!"

Because of the makeover, she goes out now with her boys, shopping and portraying a different image than one of "overwhelming motherhood." "I was feeling undone; now I feel more complete. Now I just feel better."

New babies do have first priority over everything else, especially triplets! But that doesn't mean they become your only priority—if Mom's not happy, she can't give enough of herself to anyone else. When you are happy, energized, and confident, you share these traits with your children. So one of the biggest reasons women give up on beauty—their children—is actually the reason to fight even harder to regain it.

Giving to everyone except ourselves is not a character flaw or a weakness. Women are very strong, with a large "coping" capacity.

Women show their strength in the care and help they give to others. Giving to others feels rewarding and unselfish. Just remember, there must be a balance.

Selfish or Self-Loving

Children absorb the values of their parents. You may have been taught not to be selfish. Selfishness is bad behavior. Being selfish is taking the last piece of cake, without asking if someone else would like it, or not sharing your toys. Teenagers are often accused of being self-centered. You may have been accused of this growing up because you used up all the hot water in the shower, or you stayed out too late, without bothering to call home, or you left your clothes on the floor for your mom to pick up.

Memories of being selfish can influence our thinking as adults. We equate spending time on ourselves or caring for our well-being with being selfish. What do you think about the word *self-indulgence*? Is it wrong to be self-indulgent? I used to think so, especially when I became a mother. Indulging myself with shopping, reading a book, or getting a haircut was taking money or time away from my children. Self-indulgence translated to being a "bad mother."

✿ LAURA'S STORY

Like many moms, I spent countless hours on the sidelines of my kids' sports activities. With my sons, it was their three-hour-per-night gymnastics practices. Each night I took a look around at all the other moms sitting on the bench gaining weight along with me as we continued marching up to the snack table. We passed the time being so dutiful. While the team was getting more fit and muscular, I was flirting with the two-hundred-pound mark on the bathroom scale. But after my epiphany, I realized that I couldn't continue like that. It suddenly dawned on me that the boys had a coach, and I certainly did not need to sideline coach along with him. I got up from the bleachers and changed. I started dropping the boys off at gymnastics and then headed to the gym. I applauded at their meets and celebrated their progress and medals. They started congratulating their newly fit mom.

If you think as I did, then it's time for a change. Being selfish when your actions are self-loving is a positive behavior, for it demonstrates that you are important. I'm not saying you should be a narcissist, but neither should you put yourself last. Love yourself enough to be self-confident. Start thinking you deserve the same attention you give to others.

You've heard the phrase "You must take care of yourself because no one else will do it for you." I reworked that phrase in my mind: "You must take care of yourself because nobody else is *responsible* to do it for you." Owning responsibility for your life is healthy. You are responsible for breathing, eating, sleeping, or making enough money to live. But that duty must extend to your emotional needs. Include yourself in the role of caring, loving, and nurturing. Sacrificing yourself and putting others first will leave you hurt, angry, lonely, and bitter. Martyrdom is not attractive and not rewarding.

STEFANI'S STORY

Stefani loved her husband and all of her six children. To her, motherhood is a blessing. Her epiphany moment came when her nineteen-year-old daughter told her she needed to stop dressing like "such a Mom." That was it for Stefani. She instantly started shopping at the Gap and Express. Next came the haircut and makeup change. She wrote to me for a makeover and after hearing her plea to escape from Frumpsville, I scooped her into my chair.

During her makeover while I was coloring her hair, I congratulated her on taking time for herself. Stefani immediately welled up with tears, her face turning beet red. "I don't know why, but doing things for myself seems selfish." Intellectually, Stefani knew she deserved to take care of herself, but caring for six put her in the "rut of self-sacrifice." She pushed on through her makeover and has continued to take care of herself with regular hair color and cuts. The makeover has brought on a new spark in Stefani. "My daughter who scolded me for being such a Mom calls me a 'hottie' now."

Like many Moms and self-sacrificing wives, Stefani felt that caring for herself was taking away from her family and was therefore selfish. If you think this way, ask yourself what kind of example you are setting for your children. Are you teaching them that you are not important? The best lesson you can pass on to your children is self-respect. Consider very carefully what you role model to others, especially your sons and daughters.

Change Your Words, Change Your Mind

Actions of caring for your well-being should never be thought of as selfish. Change the word *selfish* to *self-respecting*. Caring for yourself is the epitome of self-respect. People are drawn to people who like and respect themselves. Your goal is to give yourself permission to like and appreciate yourself as well as the time and attention you would give a loved one or your lover.

Here are some excellent inspirational words containing the word *self* and their meanings. Whenever you think that your actions of caring for yourself are selfish, remind yourself of this list:

Self-appointed—designated so by oneself, not authorized by another

Self-aware—conscious of one's character, feelings, motives, and so on

Self-esteem—good opinion of oneself

Self-made—successful by one's own effort

Self-help—theory that individuals should provide for their own support and improvement

Self-respect is a very powerful word and should be your constant goal. Synonyms for self-respect are *dignity, pride, honor, integrity,* and *self-regard.* These are characteristics you hold in high esteem for others. You must desire them for yourself.

Without self-respect or self-esteem, your self-worth will deteriorate. People with little or no self-worth believe that they do not deserve what others have. Some people don't give themselves permission because deep down they feel they don't deserve what they want.

LYNNE'S STORY

"When I left my marriage, I was at the depths of despair." Lynne Rominger had spent seven years with her husband, but really hadn't known who she was or felt good about herself. "We could never have a good relationship because I was always worrying about everyone else and what they thought." So at the time of her divorce, she and her ex-husband didn't have a positive, supportive relationship. "Because of the instability, I felt ugly and stupid."

Even after leaving, she didn't feel worthy of having anything. Lynne took nothing with her except some bills and their two children and moved in with her parents.

Within a few weeks, she started feeling ill, really nauseated. Lynne was pregnant again. But not only with one child—she was expecting twins. In August 1998, she gave birth to twin girls. Now she was alone with four children to care for.

Though she was free from the instability in the relationship, her emotional scars and guilt were deep. "I felt awful about myself. I had no self-esteem. My job as a freelance writer allowed me to hide at home for the most part, conducting interviews over the phone." She seldom put on any makeup. Her hair was prematurely graying from all the stress, and she never wore anything but Hanes sweats—because she'd gained so much weight, tipping the scales at 230 pounds. "I ached everywhere—throughout my bones and certainly my heart. Echoing in the back of my mind as I struggled to provide for four little mouths was my own self-doubt about ever having a strong relationship." All I could think was, "No man will ever want you with four kids! Look at you—you're disgusting." Lynne was so depressed that her doctor put her on Prozac when the twins were five months old.

Lynne had seen me on television but she still believed so little in herself that she was embarrassed to ask for a makeover or be seen on television. "I wanted to hide through the process—which I did."

Lynne's transformation began with little steps. Just making a few small changes boosted her self-esteem. She remembers first putting on a full face of makeup and getting a compliment from a passing stranger: "You're beautiful!" That positive reinforcement compelled her to do more. She began walking and losing weight. Soon, she felt good enough to pursue in-person interviews and was actually living her career instead of sitting in front of a computer screen and hiding from her job. Within a year, she was a different person emotionally and physically. She started dating again. Further into her makeover, she even braved locker rooms to interview athletes for sports stories. "Where once I couldn't look at a man because I felt so very ugly, now I asked them questions while they sat in their towels!"

Yesterday Lynne sat in sweats and hid from the world. Today, she's the author of six books and more than two hundred magazine articles. "I have more energy to give to my children because I'm happy and I don't hurt anymore."

Lynne looked toward everyone else's approval but her own. The secret to the successful recovery of her self-respect was to reconstruct it on her own. She permitted herself to feel and be important. Her self-worth was rebirthed from within.

Permission Granted

The common thread with many women is that while we may know what we want, we often look outside ourselves for the permission to pursue it. The message is simple but powerful. You don't always need to seek the permission of others. It's okay to own your own power and give yourself the permission. Give yourself the permission to hold your head up high. Go to the gym every day if you feel like it. Regard yourself as important as friends and family are. Give yourself permission to take whatever steps are necessary to look your absolute best every day . . . not just at your best friend's wedding.

Rewrite the following sentence: "I must take care of myself because nobody else is *responsible* to do it for me."

_____

_____

_____

Now, write yourself a permission slip. List at least six privileges that you will allow yourself to work toward your transformation and your new life. (Example: "Starting today, I grant myself permission to join a gym, color and cut my hair once a month, buy new shoes, etc.")

I grant myself permission to

_____

_____

_____

_____

_____

6

Putting Beauty Myths to Rest

![Stacey Ward before]

Stacey Ward before

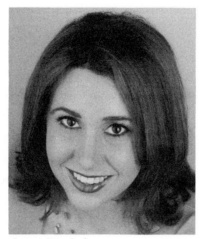

Stacey Ward after

> "Most women's magazines simply try to mold women into bigger
> and better consumers."
>
> —GLORIA STEINEM

"I need you to look at my face shape and tell me what kind of haircut will be the best," says Angela, a thirty-four-year-old mother of two toddlers and who works in the home.

"My problem is I have a high forehead, so I need a style with bangs," declares Rachel, an accountant in her fifties.

"I have a really round face so whatever you do, make me look thinner!" suggests Donna, forty-two years old and reentering the workforce after fifteen years of raising her children.

Nearly every woman I have the privilege of consulting with could write her own book on all of her beauty "issues." I like to call them *beauty myths*. *Webster's* defines the word *myth* as a widely used but false notion. Putting these beauty myths to rest will give you a clearer view of your own beauty and allow you the freedom to achieve a new you.

When I set out to work in the salon business, my desire was to use my hands and "decorate" women just like an artistic florist works with flowers or a baker creates beautiful cakes. Working with my hands was my passion. I wanted to create art and beauty with human canvases. In my early days, I believed talented hands would make an accomplished hairstylist and makeup artist. What I have since learned is that before I can re-create a woman's appearance I must help her rearrange the way she thinks about herself.

Somehow I had to find a way to dispel the myths—myths that some women have believed in since they were children or teenagers. The first step in a magical makeover is to transform the person on the *inside*. This is part of the mental makeover process—a beauty myth makeover. Until this phase is accomplished, making positive changes on the outside may feel awkward or uncomfortable when a woman looks in the mirror.

How Are Myths Created?

Myths are created during a lifetime. They are introduced to us at a young age by family members, especially mothers. Some examples follow.

"Oh goodness, you inherited my big nose."

The daughter may or may not have a big nose but she looks like her mother. Mom may be just wanting to bond with her daughter by pointing out a resemblance. Unfortunately, the daughter grows up and declares that her hair must be cut a certain way to hide her big nose after reading "Hairstyles for Big Noses" in a fashion magazine.

"I don't look good without my bangs."

A large percentage of women think they need bangs simply because they have always had bangs. Mothers tend to cut bangs on their little girls so the hair won't be in their eyes. The bangs remain for the rest of the daughter's life. When exposing the forehead, the adult woman feels naked and uncomfortable even though she may look fabulous with a better balance to her face.

Beauty professionals also help create myths. Sometimes my clients stick to the opinion and advice of a former hairstylist or makeup artist, as in the following examples.

"My last stylist said my face is too long to have layers cut around my face."

Very few women have face shapes that are so out of balance that they need special consideration. I find the majority of women have an oval-shaped face and can choose from several flattering haircuts and styles.

"My hair is too fine to style without getting a perm."

Be careful to consider that sometimes recommendations are suggested to promote increased spending on salon services. Perms are not always the answer for fine hair. Talk to a stylist you know and trust.

"I can't wear blue-based lipstick because a makeup artist told me I had a yellow skin tone."

There are plenty of ways to color-balance skin tones so that you may enjoy your favorite colors. You just need to know how.

Spouses and boyfriends can create beauty myths, too!

"Girls look better in long hair."

Traditionally, young girls are forced into long hair to differentiate them from little boys. I have many dads in my salon carefully supervising how much I cut off their daughter's hair. I believe that short hair can be as attractive, especially if a woman has other appealing attributes. (Men certainly notice women such as Halle Berry, Jamie Lee Curtis, Sharon Stone, and so on.)

"My boyfriend doesn't like it when I wear makeup!"

His negative comments about cosmetics might have to do with his past experience with other women. Maybe he had a girlfriend or sister who wore too much makeup. Perhaps he feels that makeup puts a barrier between him and you; that is, messy kissing and smears on his clothes. Using makeup with a natural application will change his mind, but regardless, you should use cosmetics that make *you* feel good.

Media Mythology

Magazine mythology and other beauty advice can really throw you into constant worry and a belief in false notions. Think of all the articles you have read pointing out every kind of beauty dilemma. It's an information jungle out there. Read the articles with a keen eye and common sense. Remember that the editors are presenting information for a very diverse readership. You shouldn't try to plug yourself in to every situation they are warning you about. Use your instincts and judgment to fend off the tendency to panic about everything you read.

STACEY'S STORY

Ever since college Stacey Ward believed blond was better. She carried that look into her profession as services manager for the Sacramento Visitors Bureau. It wasn't long after beginning the job when Stacey felt it was time for a more professional, sophisticated, and mature look as she represented the capital city of California to conventioneers. When she came into my salon for her makeover, I first noticed her large, dark auburn eyes. She brought with her a picture of a dark-eyed and dark-haired beauty, actress Rene Russo. I knew Stacey was on the right track. We set out on a radical change—and said good-bye to her waist-long curly blond hair. A hair color change also required a makeup change. Stacey's husband was terrified about the changes, but she was determined to follow her instincts.

The result was amazing. Her new deep auburn hair made her face come alive. Stacey saw others were noticing. "My new look makes me feel more confident, polished, and presentable. No longer do I look too young for my job. I've noticed a big difference in how clients perceive me." The shorter and darker hair was the perfect frame for the fresh, creamy complexion of her sweetheart face. New and darker elegantly shaped brows made those beautiful eyes stand out. Stacey is thrilled with the results. "The new makeup has made a huge change. I feel much more confident when I make presentations to clients." And her hubby has changed his doubting mind. "My husband is thrilled. I look totally different. I am very glad I had the makeover."

The new look has other benefits as well. It's more convenient. "It used to take me an hour and a half to deal with my waist-long hair. Now it takes about twenty-five minutes." Now that she has no more self-conscious worries about her appearance, Stacey is visiting the gym more often. She thanks Rene Russo for the inspiration!

Putting Common Beauty Myths to Rest

Okay, let's tap in to some of that common sense and slay some beauty dragons!

"There is only one haircut that is good with my face shape."
If that were true, then all the hair changes you see on actresses, models, and celebrities are working against them most of the time. Think of the variety you see on famous glamorous women. Can you

imagine Meryl Streep or Meg Ryan in only one hairstyle? The reason they pull off various styles is because:

- Most faces are usually oval so the choices are vast.
- The celebrities' confidence shines through so we accept the hairstyle.

Don't worry about your face shape. Select a style you like and hold your head up high.

"I'm overweight. I need a hairstyle that will make me look thinner."
When women make the observation that they are carrying extra pounds, they hope a hairstyle change will take the attention off their weight, thus boosting their self-esteem. My experience has taught me that if a woman feels she is heavy, a haircut change will not magically change her view of her body. If you want to be thinner, let's redesign your body, not just your haircut.

"Those aren't my colors; I am a winter (fall, spring, or summer)."
The theory of restricting yourself to a color palette started in the early 1980s and is still practiced today. In my modeling days I never experienced an art director or photographer requesting a model based on her color palette in order to wear the red Dior dress on a magazine cover. Wear colors that make you feel confident and that you love. Then learn to control the balance with your makeup.

"I'm too old to wear my hair long."
Women flock to salons to color the gray in their hair to defy age. They also tend to perm and crop their hair shorter as they get older, creating the "retired" look. Go for the look you love whether it is long, medium, or short. I believe women are attracted to shorter hair as they mature because they don't want to spend a lot of time styling their hair. My message is to give yourself the quality time you deserve.

"It's too late to get in shape."

I used to believe that, too, but not anymore. Your body can be transformed at any age no matter how large or soft. Never talk yourself out of the thrill of reshaping your figure.

"I'm short, so I need a hairstyle with height."

Fluffing your hair up on top of your head may achieve a half inch of height but a dated 1980s haircut will diminish your stature because it will make you look old-fashioned. Never trade in a great-looking hairstyle for a bad one because you believe the style will make you look taller. It's not a good trade-off. Being taller isn't as important as looking current and terrific.

Shelving Your Book of Beauty Mythology

How many of these myths made you smile because you shared the experience? You may have heard your own voice as you read through the list. To proceed to the next exciting section of this book—designing the real you—it is absolutely imperative that you wipe away your own personal beauty myths. It's time for your mythology book to be permanently placed on the shelf.

Makeover Action Plan: Banish Your Beauty Myths

On the following lines, write down every negative comment you have heard about your appearance. Try to write down who created the myth as well as how old you were when you started to believe in it.

_____

_____

_____

_____

_____

_____

Read the list back to yourself. Now make a big X over the list. From here forward, imagine that your beauty slate is wiped clean with no myths, rules, or restrictions. Your image and transformation will begin instead with your desire to look your absolute best. Without any boundaries and preconceived notions, you may design and choose how you want to look and the image you want to project. If you don't know how to accomplish this yet, don't worry. I will show you and teach you every positive beauty technique and secret that I know. From now on I will encourage you to think of beauty and the changes you will make only in a positive nature. It's not about what you can't do, or shouldn't wear, it's all about what the possibilities are and what you can accomplish.

7

Leap of Faith

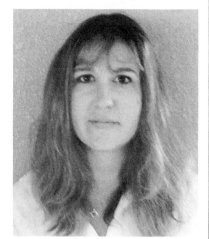

Kellene Kozub before

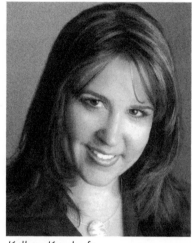

Kellene Kozub after

"There comes a moment when you have to stop revving up the car and shove it into gear."

— David Mahoney

My parents gave me the greatest gift I could ever receive: faith in myself. When I was growing up, the theme in our household was "You can do it." They would always say to me, "If anyone can do it, Laura, you can." I didn't realize the power of this principle until I really had to put it into action in the last decade of my life when I hit rock bottom.

At the pivotal age of forty, the "doomsday year" for many women, I was facing a mountain of debt I couldn't scale and was advised by my accountant to file for bankruptcy. It seemed at the time the only way of saving the home I needed to raise my boys. While sitting before the judge in the bankruptcy court, I kept hearing my parents' words over and over again in my head, "If anyone can do it, Laura, you can!" I realized that morally I could never walk away from the debts that I owed. I had the bankruptcy proceedings halted. For the next six years, I worked six and sometimes seven days a week, to clear all outstanding bills, keep my house, and rebuild my single salon. I took my parents' advice over the advice of a financial professional and did what I knew was the right thing to do. Through faith in myself, I took the high road.

Definitions of Faith

You don't need to have money, or to be a fitness or beauty expert to succeed in transforming your mind, body, and spirit—but you must have dreams, goals, and determination. Most important, you must have faith. Without faith, there is no reason to believe that you can accomplish your goal or that your goal will bring you fulfillment. Religious faith is very important for millions of people around the world. In this book I wish to emphasize *personal faith*. Focus carefully on these definitions of faith:

- Complete trust or confidence
- A firm belief, especially without logic or proof
- A duty or commitment to fulfill a trust or a promise

Three Leaps of Faith

The power of these three meanings when applied to your own life will give you the ability to succeed in anything you do. Think of applying these definitions to yourself. These foundations of faith will empower your success in your life-changing transformation. I refer to them as the three Leaps of Faith:

- Faith in Yourself (complete trust and confidence)
- Faith in the Power of Beauty (firm belief, especially without logic or proof)
- In Good Faith (duty or commitment to fulfill a trust or promise)

FAITH IN YOURSELF

Almost every woman I know who has experienced a successful makeover has learned that you have to take the first step. You have to dare. You have to act. You have to take a risk. The only thing that will keep you from expressing the faith within is fear. You may fear the disapproval of others when you communicate to them that you are on a self-improvement plan. You may fear the unknown.

⚘ SHARON'S STORY

Two years ago, Sharon Schneider felt her life was a mess, and she was seriously depressed. In the course of only a few months, her sister-in-law and her lifelong best friend had both died. To complicate things, she had to quit her job as a floral designer—a profession she was proficient at and loved—and could no longer drive because she was swiftly losing her sight from a genetic disorder called retinitis pigmentosa. With losing vision, the death of her loved ones, and leaving her job, it had just pushed Sharon over the edge. She felt helpless and hopeless.

All day Sharon would watch television and stuff her face. Most days, she wouldn't even shower or dress, instead choosing to stay in her nightgown. As her overall sight continued to deteriorate, Sharon deteriorated, too.

Then one day, something happened. A realization set in as Sharon sat in front of that television, all weepy and unkempt. "Although I had always been a little more low maintenance in my appearance, I loved watching Laura DuPriest's Monday Makeovers. Suddenly, I thought, I can't do this anymore. I've got to do something." She wrote me a letter requesting a makeover but never thought I'd pick an "old broad" like her—she's now in her late fifties. Well, I didn't see Sharon as an "old broad." I saw sparkling eyes and a very youthful face hidden behind a mask of sadness and despair. Together we got to work with simple steps toward change.

"Little did I know," says Sharon, "that this one letter would create such a change and that I would become inspired to remake myself in attitude as well as looks. Just because I was going blind didn't mean I wanted to look like an unmade bed to the rest of the world!" Sharon's makeover went beyond hair color and makeup. We talked about the importance of dressing up—or "getting the guy out of your closet." No more baggy sweats or boxy T-shirts (more on this in chapter 14). Even though Sharon soon may not be able to see the color of her hair, she realized other people would. "I plan on keeping the gray out forever!" Sharon's transformation has been so complete that she's now even an inspiration to other adults who are going blind. She got herself up off the couch and enrolled in the Orientation Center for the Blind, where she was voted activities director. Although most of the other women wear sweats, she feels so much better dressing up in slacks and blouses each day. "One of the ladies paid me a wonderful compliment when she told me that I had inspired her by *not* wearing baggy clothes and taking the time to fix myself up." Because of that compliment, she asked one of the teachers if she would create an extra class to teach the students about style and colors, so everyone could feel better about themselves and confident in their looks. "I try to motivate my classmates to eat better and to take a water aerobics class with me. One step at a time, we now are all going from frump to fabulous!"

Initially, Sharon had no idea whether a makeover would change her life. "I just knew I couldn't stay the way I was, a frumpy mess, wallowing in my depression over losing my eyesight. I wanted so badly to feel better about something in my life. I had to believe that if I could just take a step forward, things would get better."

Sharon stepped out in faith, not knowing that a makeover would empower her to rebuild her life. "A year later, I'm losing weight, taking the time to dress nicely each day, wearing jewelry, and getting around town by myself. Last year I sat on a couch and cried all day. I am working to help other visually impaired and blind women with self-image issues. My new career is exciting and very rewarding. I have felt the way these ladies do and I know that they, too, can overcome the self-defeating thoughts and move forward with their lives.

"Even though I'm physically losing my sight, emotionally I see clearly now; I have my life back!"

Sharon unfortunately had to contend with an extreme change in her life, losing dear ones and going blind. But once she had her epiphany, she came to terms with her life and has emerged triumphant. Isn't it interesting that when she gave up the fear about all the things she could no longer do, she started doing things she never dreamed possible. Bravo, Sharon!

My experience shows me that the timid seldom succeed in bettering their physical and emotional conditions. They are often afraid of the consequences of taking a risk. From where you sit now, chances are that making yourself over may feel risky. On the other hand, a transformation may be the greatest thing you've done in your life. What have you got to lose? Whenever you are faced with an uncertain situation that feels scary, ask yourself, "What is the worst that can happen if this doesn't work out? Will I starve? Will I go broke? Will I lose my family?" Once you mentally work through the uncertainty you will became more enthusiastic and passionate about taking a risk and being your own person. That's faith in yourself.

FAITH IN THE POWER OF BEAUTY

You may have experienced this or not. If not, your faith in the power of beauty may be a big leap. Trust me and the other women who have experienced this power. Your transformation will impact the way others positively react to you, and you will benefit greatly from the experience of putting beauty back into your life.

⁄ℬ KELLENE'S STORY

Kellene's life was going along great—better than it had gone in years. She was going to get married to a wonderful friend from her past. When they reconnected, they found that they were both struggling as single parents. They fell deeply in love and made plans to merge their families.

Soon after their engagement Kellene's daughter was diagnosed with a health problem, forcing Kellene to strictly monitor her diet. Kellene followed the same modifications to support her daughter. Like many moms, Kellene had let her body go because of the responsibilities and stress that raising four children can bring. As she changed her diet, the pounds started to come off. Even though her thoughts had been about eating for better health, the renewed confidence in how her body looked inspired her to keep going. She started tuning in to the mirror once again and decided to stay on the path toward a more slender figure on her wedding day. She never considered changing her hair and makeup prior to her makeover. She told me that she often felt frumpy but was settled in her thinking that she was fine the way she was. Or so she thought.

It took a coworker's transformation on one of my Monday Makeovers to change Kellene's mind. Kellene was awestruck by her friend's transformation and contacted me right away for her own makeover. When she saw how terrific her coworker looked, she formed a faithful belief in the power of beauty. She courageously stepped out in faith to reap the benefits of her own magical makeover.

That night, she surprised her fiancé with her new look. He was completely taken aback. Before the makeover he remarked, "I love Kellene just the way she is," and I could see in his intensity that that couldn't be more true. But Kellene had realized the secret that all the women in this book discovered—it's about doing it for you, not anybody else. So she went ahead with her dream makeover and shocked her love with her dazzling beauty. That night they celebrated over a special dinner, and the happy memories are obvious in her carefully crafted memory book. Kellene's makeover renewed her faith in herself.

"I look at things optimistically now. I no longer feel sorry for myself. Before I would crumble and fall apart when something in my life changed."

IN GOOD FAITH

For me this is the most important part—making a deal with yourself in good faith. Faith in yourself requires that you commit to making your life better. This sense of duty is a promise that you will give yourself permission to do whatever it takes to stay healthy, fit, radiant, and vital. It's about making a promise to never go back to neglecting yourself.

Since I dropped seventy-five pounds, I feel fantastic. Never a day goes by without a compliment on how trim I am from a client or acquaintance. The recognition is delightful, because losing weight is a challenge! There is usually a nice plate of tempting treats in the salon's break room. Maria, my salon's manager, is that special kind of angel who loves to take care of everyone's heart and tummy. I look and smell the temptations of cookies, muffins, and pastries. I give her praise and thanks for thinking of everyone, but I never have a single bite. I promised myself I would never return to the "eat everything" robust Laura I used to be. In good faith, I will fulfill my promise.

The good faith agreement you make with yourself should be to raise your standards of self-caring. This promise is the same as negotiating a business deal that you make in good faith. Your deal should extend for the rest of your life. It is an arrangement that nobody can negotiate but you. The beauty of being the solo player in the deal is that no one can interfere. It's all about you and the promise you make with yourself . . . in good faith.

Be Faithful

Being faithful is an admirable quality to have and one we greatly admire in others. To be faithful is to be trustworthy, loyal, and constant.

You have undoubtedly been a faithful friend or wife or mother to others. Now it's time to be faithful to another important person in your life—you.

In the pages that follow, I will rev up your engines with my best motivational tricks and inspirational stories. I will even teach you how to drive with all of my beauty how-tos. The only one who can shove you into gear is *you*, but I promise you will love the ride, you will love the journey. Have faith that when you reach your destination you will be a winner. Start your engines!

Makeover Action Plan: Your Leap of Faith to Beauty

Review the three definitions of faith and complete the following sentences for your life.

FAITH IN YOURSELF

I have had faith in myself in the past when I accomplished:

_____

_____

I have faith in myself that I can accomplish (future goal):

_____

_____

FAITH IN THE POWER OF BEAUTY

I have witnessed the power of beauty in (give example or perhaps you may fill in when finishing this book):

_____

_____

Write down your current feelings about the power of beauty as it relates to you. These feelings may be positive or negative. (Example: "I feel that if I looked more together every day that I would feel better about going to work" or "I want to have a makeover but am not really sure how it will change my life yet.")

_____

_____

_____

IN GOOD FAITH

Write a good faith agreement with yourself as if you were making an agreement with a business partner. This good faith agreement is simply a promise you make with yourself to carry out a plan. (Example: "I agree from this day forward to start taking better care of myself. I will not let others interfere with my transformation plan.")

_____

_____

_____

STEP FOUR

Your Mental Makeover

"If you want your life to be rewarding, you have to change the way you think."

—OPRAH WINFREY

8

Put On Your Ruby Slippers

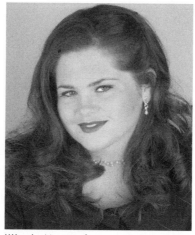

Wendy Martin before

Wendy Martin after

"Do not follow where the path may lead. Go instead where
there is no path and leave a trail."

—Muriel Strode

Not long ago, I met up with a dear friend who hadn't seen
me for a couple of years. Noticing the profound difference in my appearance, my friend wondered what had inspired me—
what secret did I discover that allowed such a total transformation in
such a short time? I poured my heart out. I told him about standing in
front of the mirror on that fateful day and receiving the dose of reality that suddenly set me back on course in my life—the path I had

lost so many years ago. I explained the special motivational technique that had always worked for me when I was young, and how I had found it again. I expressed my joy in reclaiming my power. I shared with him some of the amazing ways my life had changed as a result. As we said good-bye, I couldn't really tell if my story of transformation had made much of an impact on him.

A few days later my favorite UPS guy, Jeff, popped in the door of my salon. My assistant, Aimee, and I looked up from the client we were working on. Instead of pushing his usual cart bearing a load of shampoo and supplies, he carried only a small box. A present! It was sent by that dear friend, although I couldn't imagine what he would be sending me. Everyone urged me to open it. As I did, my eyes met with Aimee's and both of us beamed from ear to ear. Inside the box lay an exquisite pair of bright red leather Nike shoes. Aimee, who works by my side as an apprentice cosmetologist, has heard many times the story that drives my self-motivation. I finally had my own ruby slippers!

The ruby slipper story has been motivating me all my life. I can still remember how, at five years old, I found my path to success through Dorothy's story. *The Wizard of Oz* captured my imagination. I loved going through Dorothy's journey of transformation, as she went from being a lonely, frustrated little girl who felt that the answer to her problems lay somewhere else to an empowered, compassionate, and happy young woman—thanks to those red shoes. I learned the most important key to success from Glinda, the Good Witch, when she told Dorothy how to use her ruby slippers in the land of Oz.

How old were you when you saw the *Wizard of Oz* for the first time? If you were a child, you were most likely dazzled by the color, glitter, and sparkle of the famous shoes. The shoes proved to be magical when they suddenly disappeared from the Wicked Witch's feet that shriveled up under the fallen house. In the blink of an eye, they appeared instantly on Dorothy's feet, radiating a mystical power. A surprised Dorothy was told to never let anybody take the magic shoes and to guard them carefully because they would protect her.

Dorothy's adventure began with a whimsical journey down the

Yellow Brick Road to the Emerald City, to find the Wizard. She was told that this Wizard would solve her problem of finding her way back home to Kansas. She exhibited trust and faith and believed that he had the answer. Off she went.

You are probably familiar with the rest of the story. Along the way, Dorothy met the Scarecrow who thought he wasn't very smart and needed a brain. The Tin Man needed a heart, and the Cowardly Lion tearfully needed some courage. They all agreed with Dorothy's suggestion that the Wizard would have everything that they needed. Her three friends developed faith and trust, and they now believed that the Wizard would solve their problems as well. Upon arriving at the Emerald City, the Wizard presented the Scarecrow with a brain— a diploma, symbolizing education. The Tin Man received a simple clock to remind him of a ticking heart. The Tin Man didn't need a physical heart because he was already kindhearted and caring. The Lion was awarded a medal and by merely placing the medal on his chest, he gained all the bravado he needed to fuel his confidence. For Dorothy, the Wizard simply needed to provide the vehicle, but as you know, the balloon took flight without Dorothy aboard. Finally, Glinda, the Good Witch, returned to explain to Dorothy that she had had the ability all the time to use the magic of her ruby slippers to get back to Kansas. "Why didn't you tell me before?" Dorothy asked. "You needed to learn that on your own" was the reply. And sure enough, with her eyes closed, focusing on her wish to get home, with three clicks of the heels, Dorothy found herself in her own bed in Kansas.

The Power Within You

The messages in *The Wizard of Oz* are simple. Look to yourself for the answers to life's problems. Don't look past your own capabilities and believe that someone else can solve them for you. It's very tempting to travel the Yellow Brick Road in search of the Wizard—someone who will handle all of your problems and deliver you safely where you want to go. You may have set off to find a Wizard to fall in love with—and you may still be hoping this amazing person will save you.

The promise of a Wizard may come in other forms. Wizards can be gimmicks like the latest diet fad, diet pills, a workout gadget you saw on an infomercial that will make you instantly trim, or a motivational Wizard who guarantees to make you rich if you buy his books and tapes. I've had people try to make me their Wizard, as if a trip to my chair will solve all their beauty problems and change their life. But here's the deal when it comes to beauty, fitness, and harmony in your home or your bank account. Nobody can achieve success for you except you! I can design a new hairstyle, but you have to decide that you are going to get up in the morning and style it, right? You can read a new diet book, but the author of that book can't come over to your house and feed you, any more than a trainer can come over and lift the weights for you. Some of these people may be valuable mentors, but they can't do it for you. That's your responsibility.

WENDY'S STORY

The challenges and stress of adulthood started early for Wendy Martin. She said she had been a "dumpy mommy since age sixteen." Besides experiencing pregnancy at an early age Wendy developed a health condition called polycystic ovarian syndrome, which causes rapid weight gain. A devoted mom from the beginning, she gave up having a normal teenage life to concentrate on finishing high school, working, and raising her son.

As soon as I met Wendy the light in her eyes gave me clues to the strong young woman she is. She went on to reveal that she is a senior at UC Davis, and that she isn't stopping there. She hopes to go on to graduate school to pursue her studies in feminist sociology. Going after higher goals has already paid off for Wendy. It was while she was studying abroad in Italy that she went from 240 pounds to 170, a drop that took her from a size 20 to a size 11. Her secret? No car! She had to walk every day about four miles, and the jump start to her metabolism started paying off immediately. When she returned to the States, she decided to continue a disciplined walking plan and continued to lose weight. Her overall weight loss was 85 pounds over the course of a year. Her determination and strong will has sparked a new drive in her. She is enjoying the payoff of a healthier, more beautiful figure. "It was a burden, literally and figuratively, that was lifted from me. It felt freeing. It was almost like I reached who I was inside and showed it off proudly for the first time in my life."

I selected Wendy for a makeover because of her positive attitude and dedication to being a mother without giving up her dream of a higher education. I could see she was wearing her ruby slippers. Her desire for a salon makeover after her body transformation was to appear more professional. Her youthful, bright features reflect her cheerful outlook on life even after a difficult period in her teens. Her makeover transformed her into a glamorous classic, sophisticated young woman. "My makeup and hair makeover was shocking. My relatives were saying, 'Are you really Wendy?' It was very positive feedback and showed me the possibility of what can come next in my life."

Life for Wendy continues to be a challenge, as she juggles motherhood, school, health issues, and work, but she is looking forward to travel and a professional academic career. It was a joy for me to help her change her look from student to professional, so she could reach her goals of a future career. I know she will be successful at whatever she chooses. "I have a great sense of accomplishment now that I have control over my body. I am still asserting myself. It's like reowning myself. People say I am much happier. I give off more positive energy now."

Your Ruby Slippers

You were born with ruby slippers. That is, you were created with free will and therefore the ability to choose to do things. Somewhere along your path of early development, you may have had a parent or a teacher give you the very important encouragement that "nobody but you can do it." When we are young, we need encouragement for just about everything. That is how we learn to take risks. Remember when you first learned to tie your shoes? The first twenty times it was very difficult, but you were probably coached and cheered on by a parent until you mastered the simple task. How about going up the ladder to slide down the slide at the playground? Didn't your friends push you just a little with the old "you can do it" attitude. As adults, these words of encouragement can be easily forgotten when tackling adult issues. We tend to be self-defeating, because for some reason we feel that we are finished with our learning process and what we are is what we are. Some people actually believe this is as good as it's going to get. Do you go around singing, "If I only . . ."

> Was smarter?
> Had the beauty of a supermodel?
> Had more time?
> Was younger?
> Was in shape?
> Was happy?

If so, you may be following the Yellow Brick Road, searching for the Wizard. Stepping off this storybook path and slipping into your ruby slippers is the secret to your future, just as it was for Dorothy and her friends.

If I Only Had . . .

. . . A BRAIN

The Scarecrow believed he was so dumb that he couldn't even scare crows away. But immediately after he received the diploma, the Scarecrow spouted off some incredible mathematical formula proving to Dorothy and his friends that he now had a brain. The diploma was full of fancy writing but it did not give him the intelligence he had sought his entire life. What really happened was that the Scarecrow *believed* he had a brain. He had a voice of authority tell him so! The

Scarecrow had now transcended his old image of himself and discovered what was already there. He finally became intelligent when he stopped wanting and started believing he was intelligent.

The secret is not in wanting, but being. One of the most effective TV commercials came from the U.S. Army, which declared "Be All That You Can Be." Just as the Scarecrow chose to be intelligent upon presentation of a diploma, you too can choose right now to improve your life. I believe the hidden success secret is discovered by each of us in that moment when we realize that we already have the power within us to choose a healthier, happier, and more beautiful reality.

. . . A HEART

We know the Tin Man had a wonderful heart because of his kind-hearted actions and deep feelings he displayed. The Tin Man didn't believe he had a heart until the Wizard gave him a heart-shaped clock that ticked. In this new awakening, the Tin Man did more than listen to the tick tock. For the first time, he listened to the desire of his heart. Let your heart beat for *you*. Love yourself unconditionally, and know that you are worth loving.

Listen to your heart and follow your dreams and desires that have been with you since birth. You won't hear your heart beating but still you know it's there. Knowing what you truly desire is one of the keys to achievement and success.

. . . THE NERVE

"Put 'em up. Put 'em up." The breathy expression by the Cowardly Lion showed he was no longer afraid of anyone or anything. His new-found confidence emerged after the Wizard gave him his badge of courage. While the medal didn't give him courage, it did bolster his belief in himself. Before this discovery, the King of the Beasts wanted to valiantly fight every battle. He always stood by Dorothy's side and yet he failed to move forward and take a risk. He froze because he was pessimistic about his own capability to be courageous. The Cowardly Lion stopped being a cowardly pessimist as soon as he was acknowledged for the bravery he always had. Resist being a pessimist. Resist with all your might. You can't say "When I get confidence, I'll start taking care of myself." The key is to "act as if." Act as if you have all the confidence and courage in the world, even if you are shaking inside. Start your beauty program and then you will gain confidence *in the process*.

The word *courage* is inside the word *encouragement*. Make sure your inner voice is saying encouraging words to you. Be open to receive encouragement from the cheerleaders in your life such as your family and friends. When you let yourself believe positive things about yourself, you will have all the energy and motivation you need to take those first courageous positive steps.

You may have earned a badge of courage in the past. Pull it out and polish it. Reconnect with that inner strength you had in that moment so you can use it to face present challenges. Your self-love, self-respect, and self-empowerment will keep your badge of courage shiny and bright for others to see. Keep it polished every day. It's time to get your "nerve" on!

AIMEE'S STORY

At age fifteen, Aimee Davis ran away from her adopted parents' home struggling with daunting feelings of frustration and self-doubt. She courageously stepped out on her own at this tender age, only to end up living on the streets and trying to survive one day at a time. Eventually, Aimee married the love of her life, Sam, a police officer that she met during those tough days on the streets. Together, they started a family.

Aimee experienced her epiphany after she gained a lot of weight following the birth of her third child. Years as a mother, homemaker, and caretaker left little time for Aimee to take care of herself. "I didn't focus on me, so the weight started piling on." The old childhood feelings of self-doubt started to return. Aimee decided to gather up her courage once again and set out to reclaim herself. She started a diet and exercise program and decided to pursue a career in the salon business.

She entered the Northern California Cosmetology Apprenticeship Program and was sent to my salon for training. "I was so intimidated when I walked in and saw the beautiful, thin female employees and the Laura DuPriest name on every product that I got up to leave. When my hand reached the door, the receptionist called my name and I whispered 'Oh, shoot' to myself," Aimee told me later. Mustering up the courage to stay and take a risk was one of the best decisions she has ever made. She was hired on the spot.

Aimee has been invaluable to me in assisting with the Monday Makeovers. Her cheerful attitude and exceptional talent has reassured our makeover candidates that they were in good hands. Aimee told me that working on makeovers led to her own makeover. "I would see the self-esteem soar for women after their transformations. It brought me great joy to know I had an impact on their lives. During those glorious moments I realized this was more than a job." Aimee was reassured that she was in the right profession. The exciting positive reactions from women week after week made Aimee work even harder on strengthening her own self-esteem and personal beauty care. "I want to shine as a light for other women and make them feel like they can achieve anything," Aimee said. She truly is a beacon of hope and an example of that "ruby slippers" courage.

Stealing Your Ruby Slippers

The secret of your future is hidden in every step you take in those slippers. It is in your daily routine, your habits to take care of yourself. Ruby slippers represent self-empowerment. Never underestimate the power of your shoes, the power that you have to change, grow, and improve. Remember what happens when the Wicked Witch tries to take Dorothy's slippers? Her evil power couldn't budge them. They remained with Dorothy, a powerful possession. The Witch represents negativity, self-doubt, worry, and criticism from others. Never allow anyone to steal your ruby slippers from you. Dismiss the temptation to listen to negative thoughts from outsiders and keep your shoes firmly on your feet.

Click Three Times

Dorothy was perplexed, scared, and doubtful when she was told to click those heels. But she stepped out in faith. She took a risk and got what she wanted. A return to Kansas and home, no place like home.

When you want something you've never had, you've got to do something you've never done. Once you make a decision to take action, you simply need to summon the power to act on your decision. Click your heels three times. Listen to the desire in your heart, let your heart speak to your brain, and then muster up the courage to step out and change your life.

The Power of My Ruby Slippers

I never take my ruby slippers, the ones that only I can see, off my feet. I see them shine, with all their ruby energy, and I feel the power that lets *me* shine. And every day, when I go to the gym, I put on my red Nike training shoes that my friend gave me. I fly through my workouts. On days when I feel a little tired, lose my focus, or want to quit early, I look down at my red shoes, smile, and keep on going.

Makeover Action Plan: Put On Your Ruby Slippers

Several of my friends who have seen my red Nike shoes have also purchased red workout shoes. They continue to inspire all of us with a daily reminder of the power of the ruby slippers.

Lisa, another friend, keeps a pair of red high heels on her dresser to inspire herself every morning before going to work in a sales position. Aimee, my coworker, gave me a ruby slipper key chain that I hang on my rearview mirror in my car.

Inspire yourself by creating or buying a pair of ruby slippers. The charm or actual red shoes should be in a place where you see them every day.

Do It Now

Get up right now and go find something red, like a piece of red ribbon, and tie it on your keychain. This can be your reminder and inspiration until you get your own ruby slippers symbol!

LEARN FROM THE SCARECROW

The Scarecrow needed to be reminded that he had intelligence though he doubted himself. Take a moment to give yourself a diploma right now, and remind yourself that you are a smart and capable person.

List at least three areas of your life in which you are very knowledgeable and capable that are not related to your appearance (be bold and proud):

_____

_____

_____

Now let's examine where you think you stand when it comes to your capabilities about your appearance. Be honest and give yourself credit in a positive manner for what you know!

Rate yourself on a scale of 1–5:

    1 = Really need more knowledge

    2 = I know a little

    3 = I am knowledgeable

    4 = I am very knowledgeable

    5 = I am a master

My Rating Now		My Rating at the End of This Book
( )	Taking care of my skin	( )
( )	Applying makeup	( )
( )	Shaping my brows	( )
( )	Choosing an attractive hairstyle	( )
( )	Styling my hair	( )

( )	Eating healthy foods	( )
( )	Exercising effectively	( )
( )	Shopping for my wardrobe	( )

Have fun with this activity, and don't worry if you feel you need more knowledge in most areas. You'll know a lot more after reading Step 5, "Your Beauty Revealed." Once you've finished this book and are on your way to your new look, come back and rate yourself again. That will be your Beauty Intelligence Diploma! Congratulations!

LEARN FROM THE TIN MAN

Remember the Tin Man wanted to hear his heartbeat so he knew he had a heart? By writing down your desires, you will hear your heartbeat. What do you want? What's your heart's desire when it comes to making yourself over? Your life? List the things you want out of life, the things that make your heart beat faster:

_____

_____

_____

Now, number them by priority. Remember, yourself first!

The only way to accomplish what you desire is to click your own ruby slippers and make your dreams come true. One step and one desire at a time, find a way to work through your list. Never give up on your desires and dreams.

LEARN FROM THE LION

Are you holding on to fears that are keeping you in a rut? Write them down, starting with your biggest fear about changing your appearance.

_____

_____

_____

Now, recall a situation you accomplished in your past or a situation that you faced that required courage.

_____

_____

_____

By mustering up the courage to conquer that fear, you earned a medal of honor. Reminding yourself that you stepped out with courage in the past will mentally help you "polish" your medal of honor. Keep thinking of that badge of courage you've already earned to bolster your confidence in yourself. Find courage within yourself again and again; remember, three heel clicks.

9

The Gift of Time

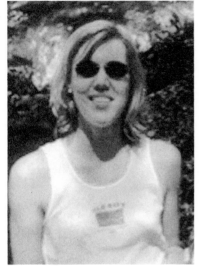

Heather Fries before

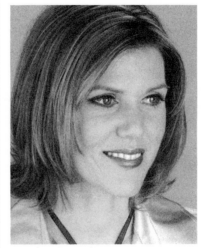

Heather Fries after

"Yesterday is a canceled check; tomorrow is a promissory note; today is the only cash you have, so spend it wisely."

—Kim Lyon

As Time Goes By

Many things get better with time—a good bottle of wine, a fine work of art, a pair of blue jeans. I've often thought, why can't time have the same effect on human beings? Time may make us wiser but plays a wicked game with our appearance. In trying to hold on to your beauty, you may be caught in a battle with time. Time seems to be in short supply for many people I know—or at least they think so.

A common complaint expressed by many women I have counseled, especially mothers, is the lack of time to take care of themselves. They are under tremendous pressure to achieve a lot in a short amount of time. I know women will sacrifice their beauty potential for an outdated style because it can be accomplished in five minutes. My mission is to convince you that the lack of time should not be your beauty adviser!

A salon is a sanctuary for women. It's a safe place to open their hearts even if they want to complain that they don't have the time to devote to their appearance; they are too busy. When a busy woman in my salon tells me that she wants to look great but doesn't have any time, I know that she's there to get beauty help and encouragement. Her feelings are valid and I understand her dilemma— **beauty versus time.**

Ladies, there are a lot of busy women out there still making time for their health and beauty! If they can do it, so can you. You have to believe you are worthy of the time. When you say that you don't have time, you are telling everyone around you that you are not important. I believe you *are* important. It's time to make a connection inside your heart and mind, so that *you* realize that you are important. It is healthy and rewarding to take care of yourself.

Time Is the Great Equalizer

For many people time is an elusive commodity, something out of their control and something only the few and the lucky seem to have. If we had more, our lives would be better. The reality about time is *we all have the same amount.* Time is the great equalizer! The day I realized that fact my life changed. I decided to make time work for me.

The Gift

Think of the time as a precious gift, instead of holding on to the belief that you were granted less time than everyone else. Every day gives us twenty-four valuable hours. Only you can decide how you will use this gift. You must take control of your time instead of allowing "time" to control your life. You get to choose how you will spend those hours. You are responsible for making them productive. Every moment—present and future—is freely bestowed upon us. Do live it. Don't waste it.

✍ HEATHER'S STORY

Time was not on Heather Fries's side. With an eleven-year-old son and a seven-year-old daughter, Heather's twenties were about motherhood, not Generation X. She married, had two children, and worked hard at a career. Heather believed a wife and mother should be committed to taking care of her family. But her loyalty was accompanied with loneliness. Loneliness because she felt no one was meeting her needs. After her marriage came to an end, Heather was feeling sad and a bit sorry for herself, and ready to blame others for her unhappiness. But she didn't.

I recognized that Heather had wisdom beyond her age when she boldly and emotionally announced in my salon one day that *she* was ready to be responsible for *her* happiness. When she turned thirty, she celebrated by declaring, "This is the year for me." This positive ball of energy finally decided to slow down and make time every day for herself. A bouncy, slender, and fair woman finally gave herself permission to be on her own priority list, for once. If she could demonstrate she could handle problems, she would send a strong, loving message to her son and daughter. "Getting my priorities in order meant taking care of myself. Being a single mom, I realized I had to be a healthy role model for my kids. They will now ask me, 'Is this a healthy food to eat?' " Heather said.

At thirty years old, she realized that her body was transforming. When her skin and metabolism changed, she made changes in her nutrition. She also saw that if she didn't start taking care of herself now, things would take their toll by age forty. She hopes that with these changes the years ahead will flow more smoothly, and she will arrive at fifty a healthy, well-balanced, and beautiful woman. "I'm a much stronger person now. I now keep my head raised when I walk and look people directly in the eye, instead of being downcast. I don't second-guess myself anymore, and I know I'm strong enough to handle anything that comes my way."

Remarried a year ago, Heather makes sure her family's days are filled with exercise, fun, academics, spirituality, and healthy nutrition. She hopes that her children will learn from her life-changing example and grow up to live balanced lives like the one she is working to create now. Heather told me, "Television is no longer a way of life for my children. Now I take them outside and play with them and go for a bike ride. We are a much more active family now. I am very proud and very happy."

Waste of Time or Gift of Time

The American workforce has found itself divided into three sections every day. Sleep. Work. Play. The eight-hour shift is no longer a reality for many workers. Several professions demand ten hours or more a day. After work and sleep the remaining hours are often filled with family responsibilities, errands, and R&R. I encourage you to make the most of the relaxation and recreation period. There is an activity in this chapter's MAP to chart how you spend your time now and how you want to spend it. For now, I want you to establish a time makeover for yourself immediately. Start today by dedicating 10 percent of each day to yourself. Ten percent of 24 hours equals 2.4 hours or roughly two and a half hours. What could you do each day with a two-and-a-half-hour block of time? Certainly, it would be enough time to tend to your appearance and exercise. And what if there was even enough time for reading, beauty naps, getting a pedicure or massage? You get the idea. Give yourself two and a half hours for *you* from the spare hours a day that exist every day. This is your gift of time.

Your Choice

Are you doubting that you can squeeze out two and a half hours just for yourself? I believe you can because I did. The secret to enjoying your gift of time is to reinvent your schedule by getting organized. It's your choice. Only you can give yourself this gift. You can fill your day with many important duties that can pump your ego and make you feel important and special but leave little or no time for yourself. Being responsible and helping others is necessary and admirable. But being a healthy and whole person means caring for yourself as much as you care for others. It is okay to be a bit selfish, but not self-centered. A big part of caring for yourself is disciplining yourself to take care of your emotional, spiritual, and physical needs. Deciding that you are worthy of that special time is taking the first step and carving out moments just for you. The next challenge is to put a time plan into action.

Multitasking

I believe you learn faster when there is a strong need to learn. As a solo parent, being both breadwinner and household manager, I know multitasking is a necessity. You are probably a multitasker already, doing laundry while making dinner. I encourage you to include simple beauty rituals with other mundane chores, like putting on a facial mask before mopping the floor. Challenge yourself with multitasking, the goal being that you will have time left over for you.

Enlisting Help

Enlist help whenever possible to get things accomplished. If you can afford to have help in the home, hire a cleaning service or someone to cut the grass once a week. An overwhelmed friend with three children reworked the household budget and cut out junk food purchases to pay for a housekeeper. Please allow other people in your household to pitch in with chores and responsibilities. Young children can perform small jobs like folding dish towels, matching up socks, and making their beds. Little ones love to help, especially if you commend them. Older children should help with chores and not just think that it will be done by "Mom the Maid." You will be helping children prepare for the real world if you get them involved with small jobs around the house. Plus, dividing up the load will give you a little extra time for yourself.

Use businesses that deliver cheaply or for free. I was amazed to find a dry-cleaning service that would pick up and drop off at my office twice a week. It was convenient and less expensive than dry cleaners in my neighborhood. Even grocery stores are starting to deliver again just like the old days. Our family shopping is now done online once a week and delivered to the door at no extra charge.

Work Time

Keeping a balance between how many hours you work and the hours you have for downtime is a tough challenge for the ever increasing number of career women. This is also true of stay-at-home wives and mothers who may feel their job fills every hour except for sleeping, not to mention the double dilemma for working mothers and single mothers who work outside the home. Economic pressure certainly may play a part in determining a long workday as does the number of children you have to take care of. Caretakers sometimes overdo it. Trying to be everything to everybody can cross over into martyrdom. Working continuously without any downtime for yourself will eventually catch up to you and take a toll on your physical and emotional health. Resentment, bitterness, and loneliness are beauty killers. I know it to be true from personal and professional experience. It is up to you to find a balance.

Set Boundaries

For balance—set boundaries, then stick to them! Examples include the following:

- Keep work at work, and do not bring it home. This is a tough one, especially for business owners, outside salespeople, and independent contractors. Making a firm decision to end work each day at a reasonable time is a healthy habit.
- If you work at home, devise a set schedule, write it down, and follow it. For wives and mothers who take care of the home, your schedule may be a split shift. Give yourself set hours off and take breaks for yourself.

Work Smarter

An invaluable suggestion from a female attorney friend, who was raising three children, was to work smarter. My initial reaction was "Yeah, right," as if anybody knew how difficult my schedule was if they didn't walk in my shoes, but still I listened. This friend always looked terrific and seemed organized and calm when she sat in my chair every three weeks to have the gray colored out of her hair. Over her shoulder I could see she was reading legal paperwork and taking care of a little business. She was making every minute count. She combined her beauty routine with her work routine.

Other clients in my chair have shown me how much they can get done while still taking care of their busy lives. My favorite example was a client who worked over sixty hours a week with her consulting firm. She would make two salon appointments for the same time, one for herself and one for her administrative assistant. She would pay for both of them so she could accomplish dictation during the ninety-minute visit. She didn't let her work schedule interfere with her appearance.

Women who stay at home bring their "homework" into the salon as well, making shopping lists, paying bills, mending or knitting.

Commute Time

If you commute by car and are the driver, you are limited in what you can accomplish. Recreational music is great company and can pick up your spirits. My favorite way to use commuting time is to catch up on the news, or listen to motivational tapes or CDs, or you can crank up the inspirational talk on the way to work, and relax with an audiobook on the way home.

If you commute by train, subway, bus, or carpool, I actually think you are luckier because you can get so many things done, such as reading a favorite book, poring over magazines or catalogs, knitting, or playing word games. I have a client who learned to speak French with her Walkman during her commute. You may also choose to accomplish job-related tasks on the way home so that when you get home, your time is yours, not the boss's.

The Lump of Clay

When it comes to time management, we're all different. Try to imagine thirty schoolchildren at their desks when the art teacher passes out thirty lumps of clay. They are told to make anything they want. Some of the children will dive right in and begin sculpting the first thing that comes to their mind: a doll, a fish, the Empire State Building, or a pretend sword. Others will pound it, massage it, squish and squeeze it, never really making anything out of it, but being busy playing with it. A few may just sit, stare, and ponder, afraid to try or just not trusting that they can make anything. As adults, the situation with time can be pretty much the same. I hope you will see that time is something you can be just as creative with as a lump of clay. Push yourself to dive right in and make something terrific with your precious gift. Start today; instead of pondering what you should do with your time, just begin doing something and you will be amazed and satisfied with the results. Try not to fall into the trap of feeling too busy, and looking busy but not getting anything accomplished. It's your lump of clay, and the wonderful revelation is that each day you get a new lump of clay to create something with all over again!

Enjoying Your Gift

The main purpose of taking you through this adventure in time management is to start you thinking that you do have control over time and that it must not control you. That is the only way you will enjoy life, with all of its duties, responsibilities, niceties, and passions that you have a right to experience and help others experience as well. The real point of this chapter is to convince you that you deserve to spend time on you. Undoubtedly, you are very important to your family, friends, and relatives. By taking time for yourself, you are acknowledging your importance as well. Remember, there is no expiration date on beauty, health, and personal growth.

Makeover Action Plan: Giving Yourself a Gift of Time

I have always believed that one can find the time for the things we love to do and for those we love. Women will dedicate time to a project that they find worthy of their devotion.

You can fill the spaces on your calendar day in and out with many important duties, leaving little or no time for yourself. A big part of caring for yourself is disciplining yourself to take care of your emotional, spiritual, and physical needs. Deciding that you are worthy of that special time is taking the first step in carving out moments just for you. The next challenge is to put a time plan into action. First, let's look at how you spend your time.

Using the following clock, to chart out what you are currently scheduling for yourself each day for sleeping and working (inside the home or outside). Shade in your spare time; it should be roughly eight hours. See the example.

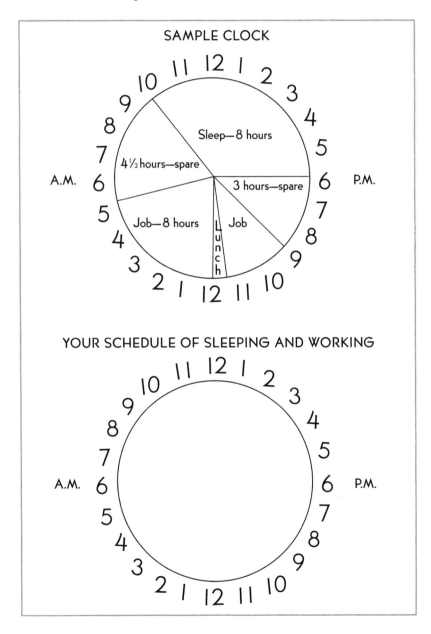

SAMPLE CLOCK

Sleep—8 hours
4 ½ hours—spare
3 hours—spare
Job—8 hours
Lunch
Job
A.M.
P.M.

YOUR SCHEDULE OF SLEEPING AND WORKING

A.M.
P.M.

The next goal is to give 10 percent of each day to yourself. Picture it as a gift, as if you had a gift certificate to spend on anything, and write down a list of what you would like to do each day for yourself. You may have a wish list with items such as taking a nap, going to yoga class, working out at the gym, reading a book for an hour, or looking at magazines.

SAMPLE WISH LIST	TIME DEDICATED
Work out	45 minutes
Read the paper/go to coffee shop	30 minutes
Bath/hair/makeup	45 minutes
Watch TV	60 minutes
Read before bed	30 minutes

It's okay to exceed your time of two and a half hours. The important point is not to reduce this precious time that you allow for yourself.

YOUR WISH LIST	TIME DEDICATED
_____	_____
_____	_____
_____	_____
_____	_____
_____	_____

Now go back over the list and number the items in order of importance. Your wish list can occur every day as long as you can fit it in with your task list. Let's talk about your task list. Write down on this list the responsibilities you must attend to other than sleep and work.

SAMPLE TASK LIST	TIME REQUIRED
Breakfast	20 minutes
Commute to work	30 minutes
Fix dinner/eat	60 minutes
Chores	45 minutes

*If you have children, add things like:

Shuttling children/school/sports	30–90 minutes
Check homework/bedtime stories	30 minutes

Write down your weekday task list.

TASK LIST	TIME REQUIRED
_____	_____
_____	_____
_____	_____
_____	_____
_____	_____

You've probably figured out the next step, blending the two lists to-gether in an eight-hour block, assuming you work eight hours and sleep eight hours, unless you don't have to work outside of the home (in that case, you may have more time during the day to accomplish your task list). Notice that the two lists have different headings marking the minutes spent. The wish list has dedicated time while the task list has time required. I purposefully directed you to fill out the wish list first because dedicating time for this list will fulfill your personal desires.

After adding up the total number of hours and minutes, see if you can accomplish both lists in your eight hours. If the answer is yes, great! You have achieved a nice balance for your spare time—in the-ory at least. If not, then you will need to get down to the business of multitasking, hiring help, or eliminating items on your task list.

Remember, at the very least you should devote 10 percent of your day to your own needs. If you simply cannot schedule 10 percent of your day for yourself during the work week, do the best that you can. Make up YOUR gift of time on your days off.

10

Mind Over Body

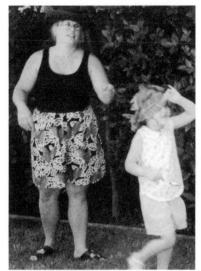

Kerry Davis before

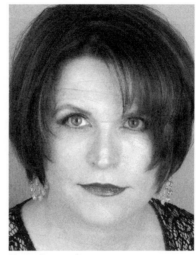

Kerry Davis after

"Once I decide to do something, I do it. I'm fearless."
—Ann M. Fudge

When people see my "before picture" they often remark, "Oh my gosh, that was you? How did you *lose* all that weight?" The question that is equally important is, how did I *gain* all that weight?

I'll never forget the painful day I finally tuned in to how much weight I had allowed myself to gain. My first and only thought was "What have I done? I now weigh 194 pounds!" I believed I was doomed to look as I did then for the rest of my life and that I would probably get larger. I went to bed depressed and sad that night. It may sound selfish and egotistical, but I didn't want to be a blob. I felt like a failure looking so sloppy and frumpy. My body would attract the same kind of looks you would give to a run-down house or a beat-up old car. I wasn't alone in my criticism. My family and close friends were beginning to look at me with that one-raised-eyebrow look of concern. "What happened to Laura the 'achieve-a-holic'? Where did her model's body go?" And, more important, "What's going on with her that she let herself go?"

It wasn't a question of where I went, or what happened. It was what I *did* that turned my once fit runway model's body into a marshmallow. I got out of bed the next day with a revelation. If I did that to my body, I could undo it. An amazing power is released when the human mind makes a decision. I chose to be healthy. Motivated to action, I went to the bookstore, but I wasn't sure what I was looking for. A diet book? A fitness book? A self-help book? I only knew I had to do something different. I had been going to the gym regularly for the past five years, resulting in a constant weight gain. Obviously, I was doing something wrong. Dreadfully wrong.

Instead of heading directly to the books, I wandered over to the magazine rack and gazed at the gorgeous bodies in the women's fitness magazines. Pictured was an array of nineteen-year-old supermodels posing in bikinis. Headlines screamed instant fixes. "Thin Thighs in Two Weeks" or "Flat Abs in Only 5 Minutes a Day." These magazines usually ended up on my coffee table while I lay on the couch feeling more depressed after looking at the picture-perfect bodies. My gaze left the ladies section and drifted over to the men's fitness magazines. Bodybuilding has always fascinated me. One magazine caught my eye because it featured a man and woman whose physiques were beautiful without being grotesquely muscular. Inside the magazine were before and after photos of men and woman who had started weight training. I had just seen the movie *Terminator 2* with Linda Hamilton. Remember the scene when she does pull-ups in the hospital? That amazed me! She and I are the same age, and her body was fit, slender, strong, and beautiful. In listening to a television interview, I learned that Linda trained with weights to prepare for that part. I had feared that weight lifting would make you big and burly with veins popping out all over the place. Perhaps I was wrong. I grabbed the magazine and went home.

Over the course of the next two weeks I became a sponge, soaking up everything I could read on bodybuilding, nutrition, aerobics, and conditioning. What I am going to teach you in this chapter will be the first step in a plan that is especially designed for busy women like you. My method of fitness and nutrition is not the only one on the market, but it is the one I know works for me and many others I have counseled and trained. I encourage you to take from me what will work for you and continue to educate yourself on nutrition and body fitness. Keep it simple and be consistent to develop a new way of life.

Heads Up

The pathway to a beautiful, healthy, and fit body starts in your head. No secret diet, no gimmicks or tricks will last a lifetime. Not quick fixes but lifelong solutions. The secret to having a beautiful body is to regain control over what you put in your mouth and motivate yourself to exercise without quitting. If you have started and stopped diets and exercise programs, don't worry. You are not alone. Many of us have failed at the weight game because we want to believe that there is a trick to eating whatever we want while staying trim. We may wish we could have a fit body and still be a couch potato. I want you to take those two dreams and put them in a box up on an imaginary shelf next to the "win the lottery" box. Call that shelf the impossible-dream shelf.

If you can put magic diet pills or miracle substitutes for exercise in that box, you will be taking the first and most important step to your new beautiful body. Later in this book, I'm going to show you how to get off the diet merry-go-round, get off the couch, and develop a new healthy code of behavior that will last for the rest of your life. But first, we have to cross some wires in your brain to rewire your thinking. **Your mind has control over your body.** Until you clearly understand this concept and believe it, you will be destined to flounder without a victory over your weight and fitness battle.

⅓ KERRY'S STORY

"I figured that since no one was seeing me naked, it didn't matter what I looked like." Kerry Davis let herself go after a series of negative events, including the end of difficult relationship with a partner who had complained she wasn't thin enough—even though she was a size 4! Full of doubt about her self-worth, and feeling less than feminine, Kerry stepped out of her body-conscious Southern California lifestyle and stepped into a sedentary lifestyle. But Kerry is a smart woman, and she knew she had to find a way out to get back into living with regular exercise and good nutrition.

While watching a Demi Moore movie, Kerry had a lightbulb moment. "Hey, wait a minute. We're the same age. Why don't I look like that?" That was the beginning of the end of her hibernation where she avoided makeup and attractive clothes. At a size 18, Kerry was determined to lose weight. She followed low-carbohydrate diets and lost fifty-four pounds in ten months. She told me, "Ecstatic is how I feel. I am now back in control of my life. Six months into my plan I stopped calling it a diet. It is a lifestyle change. I feel confident. It's easier to deal with stress because I feel good about myself."

Kerry's back pain went away. Her cholesterol was lower and her high blood pressure under control. Now it was time to get rid of the fat clothes. "My mother told me I better hang on to the bigger clothes because she thought I would fail to keep the weight off. But I told her it's not going to happen. I won't let it. I gave away the old clothes and bought a new wardrobe. I am in charge of my life now."

Kerry redefined her ideal for herself, not to please others. She learned to accept and appreciate her beautifully muscular body. She says "I'm a dandelion, not a willow." She may not be following anyone else's ideal, but she is certainly an ideal example of taking care of yourself because you love who you are.

What's My Motivation?

What drives one person to work out at the gym at 5 A.M. three times a week and another to ignore exercise altogether even though they can tell you the benefits of exercise? What motivates a person to exercise every day? There are a million reasons. Tour de France champion Lance Armstrong was motivated to work harder and ride faster on his bicycle after he was diagnosed with cancer. Not everyone has such a dramatic threat to motivate them. But I believe Armstrong's story is inspiring for everyone. We may take a second look at ourselves and ask, "Why am I still sitting around doing nothing?"

Obesity in the United States is an epidemic. The most recent figures from the Centers for Disease Control and Prevention show that 65 percent of U.S. adults—or 129.6 million people—are either overweight or obese. It isn't hard to notice that the "full figure" department in most clothing stores is growing while the sections carrying sizes 6–12 are shrinking. Though we know more now about diets, health, and exercise, why are there more people than ever out of shape and overweight? I have pondered that question from my own experience and from listening to clients. The common reason is that we get so caught up in our busy schedules we lose sight of the fact that we have control over our lives. Women especially seem to be so wrapped up in chaotic schedules that they feel like programmed robots, unable to make choices. This crazy lifestyle can affect you in many ways, especially in the size, shape, and health of your body. This robotic state of being can cause you to become a fast-food, drive-through, convenience-store junkie.

You can break the bad habits. Many people know what they have to do—eat right and exercise regularly—to get into shape. **You know it.** Now you have to DO IT! I will give you the nutrition and exercise tools you will need later in the book. First, we must reset your thinking to give you the most important fitness training tool, your alert and conscious mind. It will become your personal trainer.

Change Your Mind

Over the years from behind my hairdresser's chair I have heard many common reasons shared by women who have issues with their weight. The issues are challenging, I admit, but women are smart, capable, and industrious. My challenge to you is to use your mind to overcome these challenges. That's what I mean by *mind over body*. Here are some examples.

"I don't have time to exercise."

Making time or taking time is a choice—your choice. You can choose to dedicate an hour each day to keeping your body fit and healthy.

"I don't have any willpower or discipline."

You have tremendous discipline, but perhaps you don't recognize it. Going to work every day on time, paying bills on time, washing the car, making the bed every day, taking the children to school, and cooking meals for your family show discipline. Every thing you do in your life is a form of discipline. You simply need to recognize what discipline is and apply the same dedication to taking care of your body.

"I can't afford a personal trainer."

If you can afford a library card, then you just hired a personal trainer. Train yourself in research and reading first, and believe that you can achieve the same results. Then just do it. Remember the Yellow Brick Road and the Wizard? Use your ruby slippers to go outside for a walk, ride your bike, or go to the gym. Start by going even if you don't have all the directions on what to do yet. Just get out there.

"I can't afford to go to a gym."

Exercise is free if you don't mind walking, jogging, or riding a bike outdoors. Affording a membership to a gym is not as expensive as you think. Most of us could shift the money spent on junk food and movies and spend it on a family gym membership. It will be healthy for everyone.

"I'm embarrassed going to the gym looking like this."

Are you embarrassed to go to the doctor when you are sick? Of course not. Let me reassure you that when I am at the gym and I see a new member who is on the larger side, I admire that the person made a decision to start working out. Most people in a gym are far too busy focusing on their own program to notice others.

"If I lose weight, my skin will sag and look worse."

Not necessarily. I lost seventy-five pounds and had no problems with loose skin. The body is very resilient, especially when you combine eating less with exercise.

"I've tried to lose weight and it never works."

Most diets and exercise programs work very well; the key here is the word *try*. You must do an eating program and stick to it. *Try* is a word that lacks commitment and conviction. If you failed in the past, there is always the opportunity to succeed this time. You will succeed if you change your thinking.

"I'll never be thin. My parents were fat and I've always been fat."

Many families have predispositions to higher numbers of fat cells than normal. These cases are rare, but still you may have been raised eating high-caloric meals or food loaded with fat. You can continue to live labeling yourself "The Mission Impossible" or you can change the way you eat, incorporate more exercise, and challenge your family traits. You do have a choice.

Let's face it. We can talk ourselves out of anything and everything if we want to. The mind is very powerful, so it can work for us or against us. Choose to make it work for you! You know that you want to look good, and your desire is to look gorgeous and fit from head to toe. Let's start with that desire and plug in the rest of what you learned from the ruby slippers to reveal the beautiful body that is inside you. Remember that it took three clicks of her heels for Dorothy to tap in to the power of the ruby slippers. The three clicks remind me of three concepts needed for accomplishment: a heart that gives you desire, a brain that offers you all the intelligence you need, and the courage that provides the guts to go for it!

Desire.

You've got to want a fit and healthy body with all of your heart. Why should other women all around you wear a size 8 or 10 and you be left out, wearing baggy clothes? Love yourself enough to reward your self-esteem with a gorgeous body. You deserve to feel good when you look in the mirror and reap the rewards of pride and accomplishment as well as admiration from others.

Intelligence.

You are an intelligent person. Let your desire spark your brainpower and all of your mental consciousness to control what you do to your body from this moment on. You know that you have control over everything you do. You may choose to disconnect from this responsibility at times and fool yourself into thinking that you can't control what food goes into your mouth. You may even pretend that you have no choice over your schedule, making exercise impossible. But deep down, you know that you do.

Courage.

Making the decision that you have the right to have a healthy body is the first step courageous people make. The second step is to take responsibility for your actions. Supreme courage is having the quality of tenacity and never giving up. You may have just a little shaping up to do or you may need to lose several pounds. In either case, proclaim your right to a place among the ranks of women with

Introduction

Remember the hope I promised you in the beginning of this book? Along with that hope, it is my desire to bring you knowledge to empower you to make a successful transformation in your appearance and, most important, inspiration to motivate you into action. You have already read about women just like you who overcame life's obstacles and made positive changes in their appearances and their lives. Before you dive into the beauty how-tos, prepare to be moved and uplifted by the images on the following pages of my makeover friends. I want you to realize your own potential by connecting visually with the incredible transformations of these women. Remember that they all achieved these remarkable changes without cosmetic surgery. They made the decision to change on their own.

The changes in their lives were so profound that they all wanted to share their stories with you and reveal their newfound beauty, especially the beauty they have experienced on the inside.

Colleen's salon makeover was the icing on the cake, following her body transformation that included a 285-pound weight loss! I loved her hair long, so cutting off the length was out of the question. I cut layers to frame her face, but the big makeover for Colleen's hair was the color. Her natural tone had shades of blond and needed some bleaching with rich lowlights and brighter highlights.

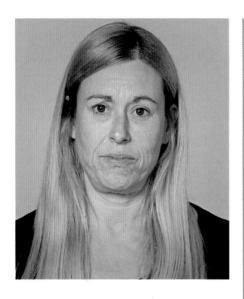

BROWS
I added an ash powder and sharpened the apex for a higher lift.

EYES
Striking white lids with black and charcoal shadow created a more dramatic look.

NOSE
To trim the end of Colleen's nose, I applied a contour shadow.

LIPS
Rocket red lipstick with a touch of clear gloss finished the look.

After losing the weight equivalent of two people, Colleen's face is firm and beautiful. Her dedication to hours of exercise revitalized her beauty and radiance without plastic surgery.

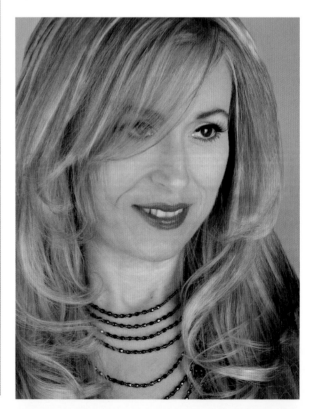

Mary's caretaking for others left little time for herself. I knew that she deserved a makeover! The challenge for Mary has always been taming her thick, coarse, and curly hair. First we deepened the color and trimmed the ends. The big secret for Mary's hair was to blow-dry it smoothly with a moisturizing leave-in conditioner.

BROWS

First I strengthened the shape with an ash brown brow powder.

EYES

I applied sparkling champagne shadow on Mary's eyelids, and a touch of walnut shadow in the crease and corners. Heavy black cake liner along upper lashes with a rich coating of mascara made her lashes look thicker. Then I accented the brow bone with an ivory frosted shadow.

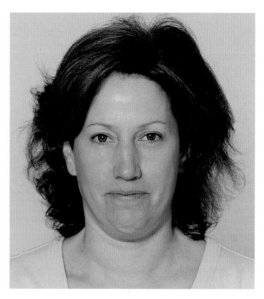

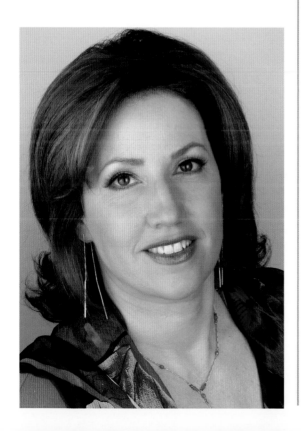

CHEEKS

Mary's cheeks were softly shaded with an apricot blush, and I kissed the upper cheekbone with a champagne-frosted blush powder.

LIPS

A glossy peach lip color accentuated Mary's perfect lips.

Before her makeover, Mary felt worn out by life's responsibilities. After losing more than thirty pounds and finding her new dazzling look, Mary's outlook on life has improved dramatically. "I hold myself in high esteem once again. My family respects me more and I love life again!"

I always knew Barbara was a natural beauty—I simply had to convince her of it. She hated her thick frizzy hair and was intently focused on that issue. She refused to see anything else. A shorter cut was easier for her to manage, especially with a straightening conditioner applied before blow-drying. Now she loves her "mane."

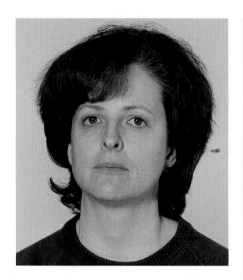

FOUNDATION

A creme-based foundation with full coverage smoothed out Barbara's freckles.

BROWS

I made her brows stronger and slightly thicker and brought them closer together with taupe brow powder.

EYES

Shadowed with walnut and velvet moss tones, Barbara's eyes really stand out.

BLUSH AND LIPS

I lightly kissed both her cheeks and lips with a warm sunset palette.

NOSE

Restructured with contour shadow from bridge to tip, Barbara's nose is leaner and longer.

When Barbara saw herself, she instantly lit up with energy. Her expression in her "after photo" tells it all. "I never thought much about outward appearance until I witnessed my own transformation. Wow!"

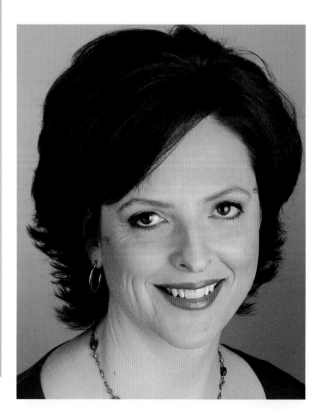

Being married with children didn't stop Susan from wanting to stake a claim in the world of beauty. I encouraged her to keep her gorgeous long hair. Susan needed multiple highlights of gold and blond to create the sexy and glamorous look she longed to have. Her hair's heavy and somewhat frizzy texture was smoothed and tamed with blow-drying and a flat iron. Layers were carved throughout her hair to reduce the weight.

FACE
Cream powder foundation was added to create a smooth and flawless palette.

BROWS
I brought Susan's brows closer together and accentuated them with a smoky brown brow powder.

EYES
Beige shadow on her lids created a dreamy look with deep copper and sable shadows to smoke up the corners.

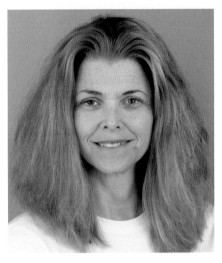

CHEEKS
I added a pale amber powdered blush to contour and lift Susan's cheekbones.

LIPS
A creamy coral lip color with a touch of gold gloss completed her look.

Susan wants to hold on to a glamorous image even though she is a fifty-year-old mom. Mission accomplished! "Going through menopause is just a little easier when you feel great about yourself!"

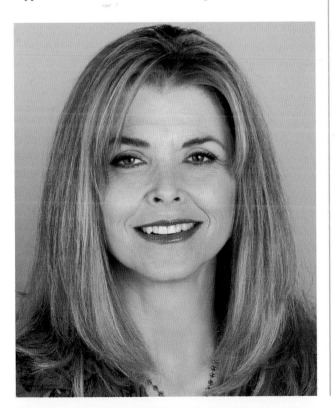

Taking pride in her appearance has always been something Lisa believes in. She enjoys being a sunny blond, so her hair was heavily highlighted and deep conditioned to give it a lot of swing. The length was preserved, but layers were added for a touch of movement.

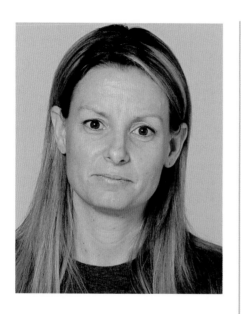

FACE

After her base foundation was applied, I lightly dusted a frosted silver powder all over her face to create a glow.

BROWS

I very softly accentuated Lisa's brows with a blond brow powder.

EYES

First I used baby blue frosted shadow on the lid with a touch of black shadow along the lash line. A shimmery navy blue shadow was added along the lower lashes.

CHEEKS

Lisa's cheeks were softly blushed with mauve powder.

LIPS

I finished with a nude pink frosted lip color that brought out her beautifully shaped lips.

Lisa enjoys tapping into her own motivation to continually take care of her health and her appearance for herself and for her family. "My joy in life is being a good example for my boys. That makes me happy."

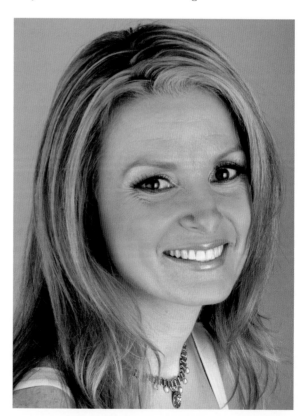

After having triplets at thirty-eight, Lynnette didn't want to look like a worn-out mom. Lynnette's natural color played up her gorgeous blue eyes, so I opted simply to use color to cover her gray hair. Her superfine hair was lightly layered to build as much volume as possible.

BROWS

I softly enhanced Lynnette's brows with an ash brow powder, especially at the apex to lift the eyebrows.

EYES

Matte beige and walnut shadow with sable liner and black mascara gave her eyes a soft, yet defined appearance.

CHEEKS

I swept a hint of mauve rose powder blush for a subtle look.

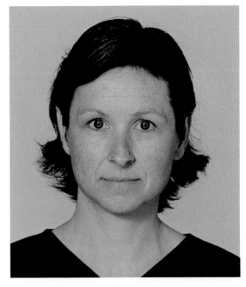

LIPS

I simply added rose lip color, as her shape was perfect.

Lynnette's makeover refreshed her radiance and energized her inner beauty. Now she glows and feels in control even with three babies underfoot. "Now I realize it's not selfish to take care of yourself. It is a need. It fuels me."

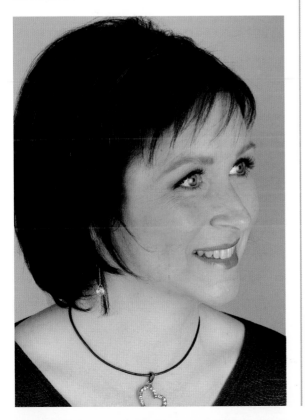

For years Lynne was told that she was ugly. Nothing could be further from the truth. I immediately saw her soft, delicate features, and creamy flawless skin. Lynne needed intensity and richness to boost the power of her natural glamour. Her hair color was restored to its natural depth and texturized with a razor for a sassy look. Lynne wanted to look confident and sexy, not shy.

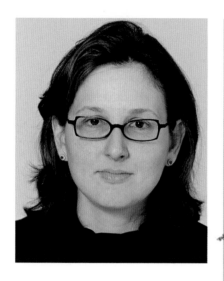

BROWS

First I strengthened Lynne's brows with a mahogany brown powder.

EYES

I swept oatmeal shadow on her lids, and walnut matte shadow was added for depth.

CHEEKS AND LIPS

Warmed up with spicy brick tones, Lynne's face comes alive.

Lynne's transformation was essentially the end of a journey back from her troubled past. Her reward for all of her hard work is her newly elevated self-esteem. "I'm the perfect representation for all those women out there who will use this book. Follow the tools set forth in these pages, and you, too, will think of yourself as better today than you were yesterday! You can do it!"

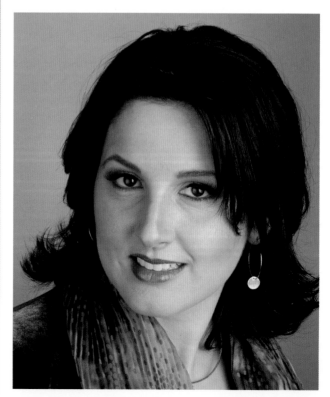

Stacey's original look, with longer, lighter hair, overpowered her natural beauty. Stacey wanted a sexy and sophisticated hairstyle that was strictly business while at work. We agreed to go for a deep auburn color and a cut that softly grazed the shoulders for movement.

FACE

Cream/powder foundation covered Stacey's freckles.

BROWS

I reshaped Stacey's brows with tweezers and smoky brown brow powder, creating a straight line to the apex.

EYES

Beige and chocolate shadow with sable liner and velvet black mascara were heavily layered.

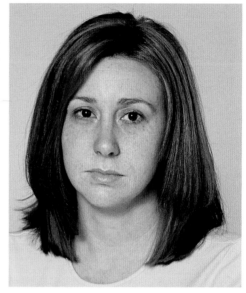

CHEEKS AND LIPS

To keep the focus on her eyes, I left her cheeks soft and peachy.

When Stacey took her makeover to the office, her coworkers gave their stamp of approval. "My confidence level shot way up! What a difference!"

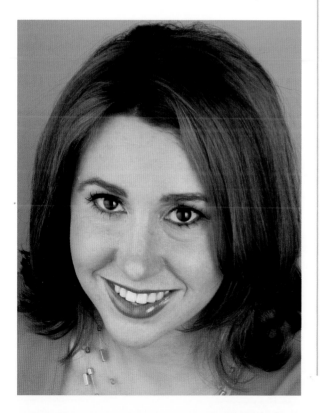

Sharon was losing her eyesight but was passionate about how others viewed her appearance. Keeping up with hiding her gray hair made this natural brunette a bit stressed. By going lighter, Sharon's upkeep would be more manageable. For her cut, I chose an easy-to-style, layered bob that she can tuck behind her ears or style forward.

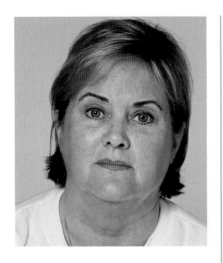

BROW

I balanced Sharon's brows with a bit of brown brow powder.

EYES

Mint and walnut shadow with deep brown liner and mascara brought out Sharon's eyes.

CHEEKS

A kiss of peach frosted blush brushed across her cheeks gave her a dewy look.

LIPS

I finished with apricot gloss over pale apricot lip color.

Sharon felt depressed and hopeless before her makeover, but now she feels like she can inspire others to have hope. "My husband loves my new blond hair. Now people say my eye color really stands out. They notice the outside, but I love how my makeover feels on the inside."

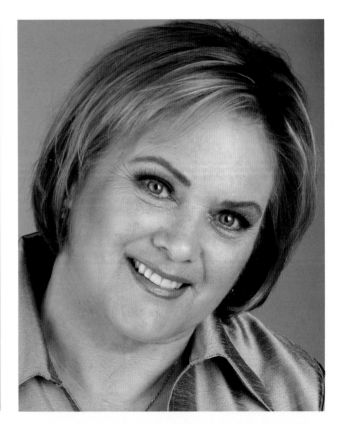

A friend's makeover inspired Kellene to explore the possibilities of her own makeover. Kellene loved her long hair and so did I, but I knew she was being washed out by too many highlights. Her natural color was accented heavily with foils, leaving threads of golden streaks. The next step was to cut extra layers at the jawline and chin to frame her face, reducing the appearance of her square jaw and putting her gorgeous dimples in the spotlight!

FACE
First I applied contour foundation to trim Kellene's nose.

BROWS
I tweezed Kellene's brows to open up the eyes and then accentuated them with chocolate brow powder.

EYES
Smoky brown shadow lifted the corners of her eyes; black liner and mascara added definition.

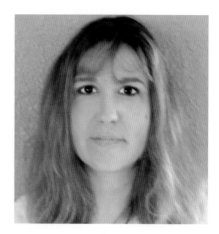

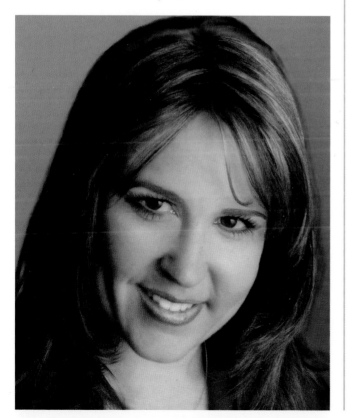

CHEEKS
I lightly dusted Kellene's cheeks with a sienna powder blush.

LIPS
I thickened her top lip with a brick lip liner and persimmon lip color and then applied a clear gloss.

When Kellene witnessed the power of a coworker's makeover, she too wanted to experience a glamorous change. Her confidence and attitude soared with her new look. "I was comfortable with the way I looked, but now . . . WOW! I feel terrific and tremendously more confident! This is the me I wanted to be!"

Wendy's makeover began with a change in her self-respect a few years ago. Making over her hair and makeup was the finishing touch. Her long flowing hair simply needed a trim to even out the shape. Her hair color was perfect and shiny.

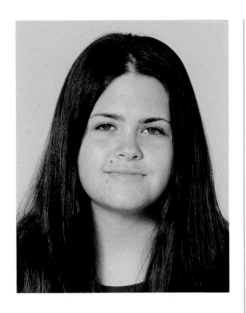

BROWS

First I tweezed Wendy's brows for a more refined shape and then accentuated them with a charcoal brow powder.

EYES

I used smoky charcoal shadow and black eyeliner with false eyelashes for a very dramatic effect.

CHEEKS

I added ruby red blush to lightly contour her cheeks.

LIPS

Ruby red lip color on Wendy's perfectly shaped lips completed the look.

Wendy lost her teenage years to motherhood and is now catching up to being pretty in her twenties. Now she looks forward to starting her career and raising her son. "No matter what happens in your life, never give up on yourself, never give up on taking care of you."

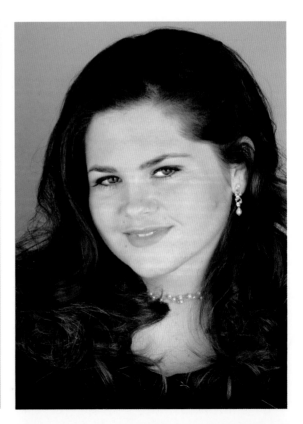

Heather wanted this year to be her time to shine. Highlights and lowlights were added to her hair for glamour. I wanted to update her haircut, steering away from bangs to layers around the face.

FACE

Heather's skin tends to be red so a mint toner was added to her foundation.

BROWS

I then used a soft ash brow powder to help pump up their intensity.

EYES

Black liner and lashes played up Heather's blue eyes.

CHEEKS

I applied a light blush under her cheek line.

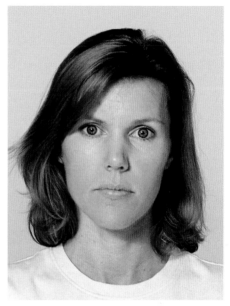

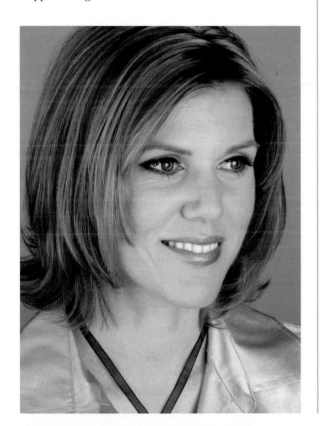

LIPS

Nude lip liner was drawn on to add fullness, and I brushed on a light rose lip color.

Heather's makeover led to a life transformation. "One of the best things you can do for yourself is finding your self-worth; then you will make the necessary changes inside and out. That's when you start really valuing yourself."

Kerry is back in the driver's seat, in control of her life after losing faith in love. Her confidence soared after shedding over fifty pounds, so I wanted to give her a makeover that emulated her new self-esteem. Kerry's hair needed a boost in color and shape. I deepened her hair with a cinnamon shade to intensify her green eye color. I then created shape around her cheekbones with a sleek, layered short cut.

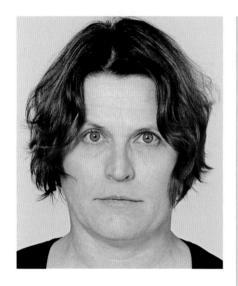

FACE
I used a cream/powder foundation with mint to reduce redness and give her skin a creamy finish.

BROWS
I thickened Kerry's brows with ash brown brow powder.

EYES
Next I used walnut and oatmeal matte shadow on her lids, with black liner and mascara to thicken her lash line.

CHEEKS
Lightly dusted with nutmeg blush, Kerry's cheekbones really stand out.

LIPS
I boosted her upper lip to balance the bottom with a maple cream lip color. Kerry lost herself after the tumble of a relationship convinced her that looking good didn't matter. Now it matters very much . . . to her! "It's about realizing that you can do it by yourself and for yourself. What better motivation can there be?"

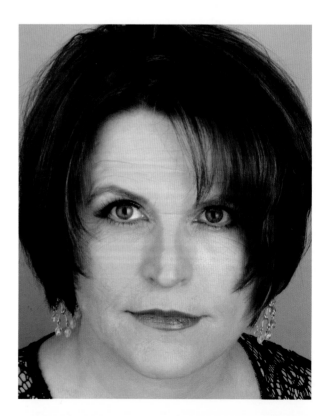

Stefani's nineteen-year-old daughter pushed her to give up looking like such a Mom! That little nudge lead Stefani to my chair begging for a fresh haircut, auburn hair color, and highlights. Her salon makeover made her spirits soar. Now Stefani shops not only with her daughter but at the same stores as well.

FACE

A cream-beige lightweight foundation was applied to even out her skin tone.

BROWS

Her brows were refined with waxing and tweezing to create a stronger angle to the apex.

EYES

Beige, plum, and black eye shadows play up her eyes for a flirty look. Mascara was layered several times to thicken her very long lashes.

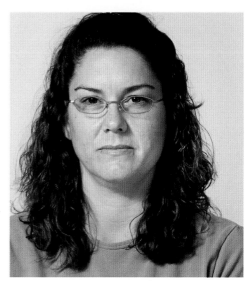

LIPS

A soft plum frost makes her lips look fuller. Stefani raises six children, but hated looking like a tired old Mom. Her transformation gave her a burst of energy she had not felt in years. "Taking care of me feels terrific!"

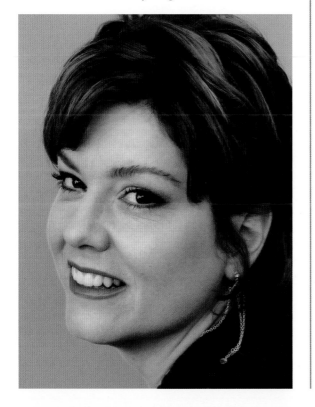

Aimee's belief in the power of her Ruby Slippers motivated her to step out and take a place in the beauty business. She wanted her makeover to be all about serious glamour.

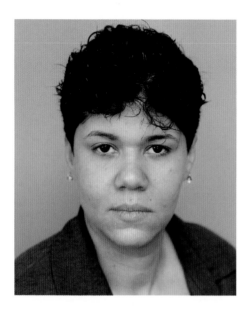

FACE
I used a gorgeous mocha shade of cream-based foundation to give her skin a creamy glow.

BROWS
Her brows were tweezed then lengthened with a charcoal brow powder.

EYES
Almond matte shadow on the lids brought them forward. I layered chocolate and purple velvet shadow in the creases to deepen and shape her eyes.

CHEEKS
Two blush shades were used to lift her cheeks, a rose matte underneath the cheek-bone and a peach frost on the cheekbone.

LIPS
A soft plum-red was used without lip liner to accentuate Aimees' near-perfect lips.

Aimee's first several weeks on the job in my salon made her an eye witness to the power of makeovers. She wanted to jump on the bandwagon and experience her own transformation. "I saw how looking and feeling beautiful changes women's lives. Now I understand why."

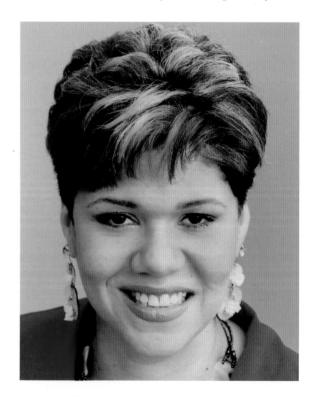

beautiful and fit bodies. As you start to put yourself back in strong physical shape, your courage will grow exponentially. You will look back and wonder what you were afraid of and why you waited so long.

Mind Over Body Truths

1. Nobody has control over my actions but me.
2. I choose the foods I eat.
3. I choose to exercise or not.
4. If I want a better body, I can take action to change it.
5. It's never too late to improve my shape.
6. Age has nothing to do with the decision to get in shape.
7. Nobody can do this for me.

Never Say Failure

The word *failure* is *not* in the vocabulary of a "mind over body thinker." Once you take responsibility and own the Mind Over Body concept, you can never fail. It's a power that never diminishes once you understand it. You may fall off your eating plan or skip exercising, but that is not failing. It's simply making a conscious decision to slack off. When this happens, your desire needs to be rekindled. You need to reconnect with your heart, acknowledge that you love yourself, and reiterate to yourself how strongly you want to achieve your body goal. Transfer those momentary feelings of failure back to desire and on to success. Failure is a word that lures us into giving up. You are far too important to give up on yourself.

Makeover Action Plan: Become a Mind Over Body Thinker

In the next section of this book, I will teach you how I successfully took control over my body after years of abusing my figure. Before you jump-start back into fitness or update your current fitness plan, take the time to reset your thinking to ensure your success. Review the mind over body truths on page 117.

Highlight or underline the truths that are already deeply ingrained in your thinking. Circle the ones that you need to affirm to yourself.

MIND OVER BODY TRUTHS

Photocopy the Mind Over Body Truths or rewrite them on a piece of paper and then make three copies of them. Place one copy on the dashboard of your car, one on your bathroom mirror, and one on your refrigerator. See them every day and read them until they become a part of your "code."

"EXCUSE ME" EXERCISE

It is normal human behavior to excuse and make excuses for obstacles that are difficult. By facing your excuses and getting them out in the open, you may be able to overcome the obstacle of controlling your body in a more active way. List your excuses or reasons why you feel you can't take control over your body. Then answer your own excuse with a positive response as if you were giving advice. Example:

I don't have time to exercise.
Response: I could make time to exercise if I stopped watching so much TV at night.

1._____
Response: _____
2._____
Response: _____
3._____
Response: _____
4._____
Response: _____
5._____

Highlight or underline the one excuse that you could easily overcome. That's the first one to tackle. After you've eliminated that excuse, move on to the next and the next, gaining confidence each time. Eventually, you will overcome even the most difficult obstacle and start enjoying the control you will have over your body.

PHOTO OPPORTUNITY

Step 1.

This may be a bit painful, but it will turn out well in the end. Have a friend or relative take a picture of you in your underwear or a swimsuit. Take a picture of your front, your backside, and your profile. Don't be embarrassed about the way you look in the pictures. This is your starting point. Keep the photos in your top dresser drawer. Over the course of the next few weeks as you begin to take control of your body, you will want to refer to your starting-point photographs for inspiration. From this point on, you will see an improvement and that will inspire you.

Step 2.

Purchase a fitness and/or bodybuilding magazine at the bookstore. Look through the magazine and tear out all the photographs of female bodies that you admire and/or want to look like. Be realistic and use common sense in selecting photos of bodies with your figure type. Put some of the pictures in your look book (refer to the look book you started in chapters 3 and 4), and others in places for an inspirational peek; for example, the fridge, your closet door, your bathroom mirror, and so on. Imagining the body you want to have is a big step in motivation. If others can build a beautiful body, then so can you!

STEP FIVE

Your Beauty Revealed

*"I have always believed that one woman's success can help
another woman's success."*

—GLORIA VANDERBILT

11

Simply Beautiful Skin

"You have only one face. Take care of it."

—ESTÉE LAUDER

When you think about it, our skin is amazing. It's water-proof, it regulates our temperature, prevents bacteria from penetrating our bodies, and regenerates and repairs itself all the time. Why, oh why, do we fret and fuss over it so much?

More often than not, my job as an esthetician is to convince my clients to stop agonizing over their skin and keep skin care simple. Skin for the most part takes care of itself in a remarkable way. The drama comes into play when bad habits or hormonal changes reek havoc on one's beautiful complexion. Take a look at the seven deadly sins we commit against our skin.

Sunbathing and Tanning.

Tanning and exposure to the sun is the number one skin abuser. Don't be fooled by tanning-booth shops that claim to sell you a safe tan. Any ultraviolet exposure will cause sun damage, and it is cumu-lative. Health clubs and salons that offer tanning booths drive me crazy, especially if they also offer facial services. It's like a doctor offering you cigarettes!

Smoking.

Smoking not only causes lip lines and smells bad, it robs your skin of the most important element it needs, oxygen, by damaging circulation. Nicotine and the other harmful chemicals in cigarette smoke constrict the small capillaries that feed skin cells nutrition. Smoking also introduces massive amounts of free radicals at the cellular level, destroying collagen and elastin. Smoking rapidly ages you.

Poor Nutrition.

I have a saying, "Eat junk food, get junky skin!" The reason that fast food and junk food show up in the skin is because you are fooled into thinking you are getting nutrition because your stomach is full and you feel satisfied. In fact, fast food may be void of the essential vitamins and minerals your skin needs to look its best.

Lack of Exercise.

If only our skin responded well to TV time, sitting at the computer, or being a couch potato, right? When the body is deprived of movement and exercise, the heart is weaker and doesn't pump as well. The circulation suffers and skin cells are slower to receive vital nutrition. Skin loses its color and glow.

Lack of Sleep.

This one is not hard for most of us to figure out because it is easy to see the signs of sleep-deprived skin. Your body needs downtime to repair and regenerate new skin cells.

Alcohol or Drug Use.

An occasional glass of wine or a cocktail is not going to ruin your skin, providing you are hydrating yourself with water. The problem with heavy consumption of alcohol is that it dilates blood vessels.

Drinkers often have red complexions and bloodshot eyes. Eventually, heavy drinking leads to liver damage, compromising the liver's ability to filter blood.

Stress.

Stress causes the blood vessels to constrict, robbing the skin cells of oxygen. Stress hormones are released and further drive blood away from the skin cells and toward the muscles. Severe stress can bring on or worsen skin conditions such as acne, eczema, or cold sores.

Before we get into the nuts and bolts of skin care or the future of your skin, make a pact with yourself to immediately adopt these new skin strategies:

- Start an exercise program. Commit to working out six days a week at least twenty minutes a day.
- Say good-bye to fast food.
- Go to bed an hour earlier than you used to. Turn off the television and computer instead of staying up.
- Invest in a full spectrum sunblock and put it on faithfully every day, even in the winter. Say no to tanning and sunbathing even on vacations. Use a sunless tanning product for color.
- Quit smoking. If you don't smoke, vow to never start.
- Slow down and de-stress. Exercise will help.
- Limit your alcohol intake to one or two drinks, or only on special occasions.

If you follow these steps, your skin will look the best it can look naturally. You are on your way to beautiful-looking skin.

Skin Care or Scare?

If you go to a department store and stroll around the circle of cosmetic counters, you are sure to get worry and frown lines. How could one possibly need all of those preparations? The misinformation and plain old drama that is created by many cosmetic companies have many women assuming they have a myriad of problems that require a fortune to fix. Don't be fooled. Taking care of your skin is very simple. The truth is, there are few topical cosmetic solutions that will dramatically change your skin, and most are not available without a doctor's prescription. The cosmetic companies want you to think you have a lot of needs so that they can sell you the solutions.

Once they point out the issues, they will intimidate you with elaborate scientific names, fancy packages, white lab coats, or fashionable smocks and high prices to lure you into the fantasy world of skin care. Let's discuss skin care myths and the facts.

MYTH: Creams can repair wrinkles.
FACT: No cream can repair a wrinkle, only diminish the appearance of one.

MYTH: Cosmetics that cost more work better.
FACT: Not necessarily true. The price of an item has more to do with packaging and marketing position. Many products with modest price tags have the same active ingredients as the high-priced ones.

MYTH: You have to use a complete skin care system for it to work.
FACT: There is no set rule. The more complicated the system, the less I believe in the credibility of the company.

MYTH: You need a different cream for the eye, the throat, and the face.
FACT: No, you don't. The skin on your face and neck, including the eye tissues, functions the same and can be treated the same, except the upper eyelids. Gravity will cause creams here to drift down into the eye, so application in this area should be light.

MYTH: Creams or eye gels can get rid of dark circles under the eyes.

FACT: No, they cannot. Dark circles are either hereditary or due to residue from eye makeup. Creams and gels cannot lighten the dark pigment under the eyes.

MYTH: Masks and creams can firm the skin.

FACT: Not so far. There are new products being tested to improve elastin production, but at this time there is no cream that can restore the firmness in your skin except for cosmetic surgery.

Keep Skin Care Simple

I find that many women either totally neglect their skin or tend to overdo it with over-the-counter skin care products. I'll be the first one to tell you that skin for the most part cleans itself. If it wasn't for makeup, pollution, and perspiration, you could keep your skin fairly clean and healthy with a washcloth and warm water. As we get older our skin may tell our age or show signs of damage. What is important for you to know about your skin is what you can do to prevent further damage and what you can do to make it look better and healthier.

Damage Prevention

Let's talk about damage prevention first. You've already pledged to stay out of the sun and to avoid cigarettes, your skin's biggest enemies. The next step is to religiously apply a full-spectrum sunblock on your face and neck every day in the morning. Never mind if you are staying indoors—even home or office lights can affect your skin. If you are headed outdoors for activities in sunlight, keep applying the sunblock every few hours. Be faithful. You'll do yourself a big service if you wear a hat and sunglasses every time you go outdoors. I can't overemphasize how much damage sun causes. Don't get lured into believing that those warm rays are healthy for you. It may feel great to have the sun on your face, but your beautiful complexion will pay the price.

Try not to worry anymore about the past and the bad habits you used to have that you now face in the mirror. You've got to go on from here. I spent nearly four years of my young life, from ages eight to twelve, living in Panama, which is on the equator. The sun shines there 365 days a year, and there was no such thing as sunblock. I have had to learn the hard way that my days in the sun are over. My focus is on treatments to make my lines and wrinkles look softer.

Antiaging Therapy

It's true that you can't buy a jar of cream and fix a wrinkle or make it disappear. Through medical advancements, physicians are getting closer to treatments that can turn back the clock, such as laser resurfacing, chemical peels, and good old facial surgery for lifting and tucking. Not everyone can afford these services, nor can you afford for life to pass you by feeling bad about the way your skin looks. You can do a fine job making over your complexion with products at home.

How do you do that? The trick to softening the appearance of lines and wrinkles is to rid the skin of the layers of dead, dry cells at the surface. It's a lot like making an old, dry piece of wood look better by sanding or buffing it. In skin care circles we use a fancier word—*exfoliation*. Exfoliation generally refers to the removal of skin cells by physical means such as rubbing the skin with a gritty substance like a scrub, but exfoliation can also refer to the removal of skin cells chemically. Chemical exfoliators such as salicylic acid or alpha hydroxy acids (AHAs) are usually gentle. Don't confuse exfoliators with peels. Peels are much more dramatic, sometimes painful, and are usually performed by a physician, sometimes an esthetician. You can exfoliate your skin by yourself at home either chemically, physically, or with a combination of the two. Combining these two methods of cellular removal is the way I teach my clients how to effectively produce beautiful results. The best part of this dual therapy is that you will feel the difference immediately, and you will see a visible improvement in two days. Here's how it works: Every night after cleansing off your makeup, apply a moisturizer with a cocktail of glycolic, lactic, and citric acid, my three favorite AHAs. Glycolic acid is particularly effective for skin due to its small molecular size. These natural fruit acids work while you sleep to break down the bonds that hold the layers of skin cells together at the surface. Imagine a wall of bricks held together with mortar. The acids loosen the mortar, so the bricks, or skin cells, are able to fall off more freely. These topmost layers of skin cells are dead and dehydrated, making skin look dull, dry, and textured. The dry skin will telegraph the wrinkles and creases of your face and neck. Once the dry layers are swept away, the cells below are newer and more hydrated, making the skin look and feel smoother.

Now comes the sweeping part, the second important step in dual exfoliation therapy. Two or three times a week after cleansing off your makeup, I want you to gently exfoliate your face and neck with a natural oatmeal-type scrub. This physical exfoliation will remove the skin cells at a faster than normal rate. The scrub you choose must be soft with fine grains. Avoid scrubs that have sharp grains. Test it on the back of your dry hand. If it feels like you are rubbing salt on your skin, avoid it on your face. It will be irritating.

Next apply your glycolic moisturizer. The idea is to loosen the layers of skin cells with an acid moisturizer, then sweep away the cells with a scrub. Once the cells are swept away, the moisturizer can penetrate even deeper, and the cycle continues. When I first came upon the idea of dual exfoliation, it was a little tricky using traditional scrubs in conjunction with glycolic acid. The freshly buffed skin became irritated when applying a dose of acid cream. In treating my own clients, I created a natural scrub with finely ground oats and almonds buffered with yerba santa to effectively exfoliate without making the skin raw. Yerba santa was then added to the glycolic acid cream, buffering the irritation commonly associated with acid treatments. I could finally offer deeper exfoliation without any irritation, resulting in beautiful skin.

Dual exfoliation at bedtime will give you an instant skin makeover. You will be impressed with the results. Your morning application of sunblock will help retard the aging process. The more consistently you execute these two vital procedures, the better your skin will look and the better you'll feel.

Other Benefits of Dual Exfoliation

I have used my dual exfoliation technique on hundreds of women. I have witnessed the positive result—not only visible improvement with antiaging clients, but those experiencing other skin dilemmas. Acne sufferers found relief and clearer complexions. The clients with oily skin and blackheads reported a decrease in both. My dry-skinned group of ladies (myself included) found that the tightness and flakiness was resolved in a day or two. One of the best improvements was for the clients who develop the stubborn bumps called milia. These unsightly, annoying lumps are trapped sebum logged just under the skin's surface. They are typical in people with oily skin who use soap or harsh cleansers, resulting in dry surface cells that block the oil glands. The milia will continue to enlarge over time and usually cannot be removed by squeezing. I have seen clients with dozens of milia covering their face making the skin look lumpy and rough-textured. Removing these bumps can be performed in a facial, but regular treatments can be expensive. My clients who incorporated the dual exfoliation therapy in their skin care routine found nearly 100 percent improvement. The combination of glycolic acid and the scrub kept the oil glands free and clear. No more stupid white bumps!

Know Your Skin Type

It's important to know what kind of skin you have so that you choose skin products wisely and use only what your skin needs.

NORMAL SKIN

Most people have normal skin, but I spend a lot of time convincing clients of that. Normal skin is generally problem free but will start to shine by noon each day. This shininess leads some people to believe that their skin is actually oily, but it's not. Try to think of these criteria in determining if you have oily or normal skin: Oily skin is usually shiny an hour after cleansing and may be accompanied by blackheads and/or acne. Normal skin will have the presence of a shine three or four hours after cleansing, but not the presence of blackheads or acne.

DRY SKIN

There is usually no mistaking dry skin. The skin feels tight almost all the time; there is never a presence of shiny skin and there may sometimes even be a flaky look to the skin. Dry skin will usually age more quickly, so those with dry skin should especially be aware of sun exposure.

OILY SKIN

Oily skin gets shiny almost immediately after midmorning and may be accompanied by acne or blackheads. Some people with oily skin don't suffer from any problems often associated with oily skin; they just have to tolerate the shine. The good news about oily skin is that it tends to age more gracefully.

SENSITIVE SKIN

Sensitive skin is usually identified as fair- to medium-toned skin that gets red or irritated due to stimulation associated with sunlight, exfoliation, cosmetic preparations, or touch. Most people with oily skin do not have sensitive skin. Oily skin tends to be fairly sturdy and does not react in a sensitive nature. Normal and dry skin can sometimes be delicate and fall into the subclassification of sensitive. People with sensitive skin usually know it. They get sunburned easily and will react adversely to harsh soaps and cosmetics.

Your Skin Care Routine

The best complexions I've seen belonged to people with two things in common: (1) good genetics and (2) consistent skin care habits.

You can't control genetics, but you can absolutely start taking care of your skin immediately. I have found that the easier it is to grasp what you are trying to accomplish with skin care, the more adaptable you will be to a routine. Many of you reading this book may have some preconceived notions about skin care or are already using a brand, a system, or prescriptions. The main question you should ask yourself is "Am I happy with the results I am getting from my present regimen?" If yes, then continue with what you are doing and by all means be consistent. If the answer is no, perhaps I can give you the help you need and deserve. Keep in mind that I am a big proponent of keeping things simple and only using products that work or make a difference. Let me run through the basics with you.

CLEANSERS

A cleanser should do just that, cleanse. I've already pointed out that for the most part, skin cleans itself in a perfect world without makeup or pollution. You should use a cleanser at night to remove makeup or "day debris," that is, pollution, dirt, oils, and perspiration. If your skin is oily with the presence of blackheads or acne, you should also cleanse in the morning as soon as you wake up. I don't believe in overstripping the skin's natural oils, so I don't promote cleansing with anything but water in the morning for the rest of you. If you did a good job of cleansing your skin the night before, then rinsing your face in the A.M. with good old H_2O works perfectly.

You may select a cleanser that works best with your skin type.

For oily skin: Use a gel liquid cleanser.
For normal skin: Use a gel or cream liquid cleanser.
For dry skin: Use a creamy cleanser that leaves your skin feeling moisturized.

For sensitive skin: Try gel or cream liquid cleansers and see how you react.

All cleansers should be easy to rinse without using a sponge or washcloth. The PH level of cleansers should range between 4.5 and 5.5, which is the PH range of your skin.

Harsh cleansers can create more problems. Don't fall into the misguided thinking that if you have oily skin or acne that you should use strong detergent-type cleansers. You may overstrip your skin of oil and cause your oil glands to overcompensate. Never use bar soap! Hard bars of soup are made from a mixture of fats and detergents. When these two ingredients are boiled together, a chemical reaction occurs, forming soap. The fats in the soap bar will leave a residue behind that may clog your pores. Try this test if you're not convinced: Rub your favorite bar of soap on a hand mirror. Now rinse under the faucet without rubbing. Look at the film on the mirror. In our family, we don't use bar soap in the bath or shower for the same reason. It leaves a film on your tub, your tile, and your skin. Yuck! No more soap!

TONERS

A toner is used to wipe the skin down after cleansing to remove any residue of makeup and the cleanser itself. I believe toners are great for this purpose, and they ensure that every trace of eye makeup around the eyes is gone. Toners are also terrific in the morning following your water cleansing. Choose a toner that is gentle enough to use around the eye area without stinging. Apply the toner with a cotton ball or pad and let it evaporate without rinsing.

MOISTURIZERS

Moisturizers should be lightweight for better absorption, colorless and odorless so as not to upset your skin's balance. You need two different moisturizers for your face. Your A.M. moisturizer should be formulated with a full spectrum sunblock. Apply it after your toner in the morning and throughout the day if needed. Your P.M. moisturizer should contain at least glycolic acid and hopefully a cocktail blend of one or two other AHAs. The acid combination will speed up exfoliation as we have discussed. Your P.M. moisturizer should be applied after your toner at bedtime. Take at least a minute to blend it in thoroughly.

SCRUBS

The only scrub I recommend is a gentle one that doesn't scratch or irritate the face. Use a scrub two or three times weekly for smoother-looking skin. You can choose to scrub in the A.M. or P.M. I like to use a scrub in the morning in the shower because it is easier to rinse off.

MASQUES, SERUM, TREATMENTS

This is where skin care can get confusing, redundant, and expensive. Suffice it to say that there are many skin care experts with many different belief systems. Consumers consume cosmetics on many different levels. You may or may not desire to venture beyond the skin care basics and make your routine more complicated and or expensive. If you do so, I would like you to know the vocabulary and theories behind these more advanced products.

Masques.

A clay-, gel-, or cream-based formula designed to treat a special skin issue such as dry or oily skin. These can be either effective or a waste of time depending on the claim. I do find the application of a weekly masque emotionally therapeutic and relaxing. If you apply a moisturizing masque immediately prior to an evening out, your makeup will go on smoother and easier.

Serum or Treatments.

These terms are interchangeable in my opinion. Serums are concentrated formulas designed, again, to tackle a certain skin problem. Most serums are formulated to fight aging, either for wrinkle therapy or dark spots. I have found that most bottles that are labeled with the word *serum* are overpriced for the results they deliver. Use your common sense and shop wisely. If the product does not deliver the results promised, don't waste your time using it.

I would prefer that you grasp the essential routine I'm about to outline and proceed cautiously to the next level of skin care, which includes the more exotic preparations. If you discover a new product that works well for you, use it in addition to your primary skin care routine. Try to avoid bringing home a huge skin care system that you might not be able to fit into your day. It's better to start a little at a time to develop a consistent habit.

Daily Skin Care Plan

OILY SKIN

A.M. Cleanse face with cleanser. **P.M.** Cleanse with cleanser.

Wipe down skin with toner. Wipe down skin with toner.

Apply oil-free moisturizer Apply AHA moisturizer.
with sunblock.

* Three times a week, use a scrub after cleansing in the A.M. or P.M.

NORMAL SKIN

A.M. Cleanse face with cleanser **P.M.** Cleanse with cleanser.
or water.

Wipe down skin with toner. Wipe down skin with toner.

Apply moisturizer with Apply AHA moisturizer.
sunblock.

* Three times a week, use a scrub after cleansing in the A.M. or P.M.

DRY SKIN

A.M. Cleanse face with cleanser **P.M.** Cleanse with cleanser.
or water.

Wipe down skin with toner. Wipe down skin with toner.

Apply moisturizer with Apply AHA moisturizer.
sunblock; add more during
the day if needed.

* Three times a week or more, use a scrub after cleansing in the A.M. or P.M.

Getting in the swing of a regular skin care routine will serve you well—you'll see and feel a difference. Remember that consistency is the best strategy when it comes to results. Even on my lazy nights, I always remove my makeup with a cleanser and always apply my glycolic moisturizer.

Special Needs

Even when you get your skin in good order, you may have an occasional skin crisis. Don't let your once-a-month pimple get you down, or worry about waking with "allergy" eyes. Temporary problems blow over quickly and usually aren't as noticeable as we think. Keep your chin up and keep smiling. Here are some quick tips for emergencies.

QUICK TIPS

For Puffy and Red Eyes

- Soak two chamomile tea bags in cold water. Blot them on a towel and apply them to your eyes while lying down for five minutes.
- Spoons in the freezer: Keep metal spoons in your freezer. Place the bowl of the spoon over your eyelid or below the eye on the upper cheek area. Presto! The swelling goes down in just a minute or two.

To Attack a Blemish

Grind up an aspirin tablet in a teaspoon and add a drop or two of water to make a paste. Dab a small amount directly on the blemish at night. It will be much calmer in the morning.

To Ease Redness from a Blemish

Put a drop of eyedrops that reduce redness on a Q-tip and dab it on the blemish. This will help reduce the redness immediately.

Simply Beautiful Skin

You can make skin care as complicated or as simple as you want. My success stories with my clients resulted from taking the simple approach. Stop buying in to the myths at the cosmetic counter. Avoid spending money just to get a new jar of magic. Loading up on too many products can irritate and cause breakouts. Keep it simple. Here's a review of my Six Top Tricks for Beautiful Skin:

- Cleanse thoroughly with a gentle gel or creme cleanser every night before bed. Remove all makeup, especially eyeliners and mascara.
- Apply a grease-free moisturizer with glycolic acid.
- Apply sunblock moisturizer every morning faithfully over face, neck, and chest.
- Exfoliate with a gentle scrub two to three times a week.
- Drink lots of water and eat nutritious food every day.
- Avoid sun exposure, tanning booths, and smoking.

Advanced Help

When it comes to your face, take advanced problems seriously and see your medical professional. Dermatologists are professionals trained to solve consistent acne problems as well as allergies, sensitivities, moles, and lesions. Salons and cosmetic counters have their place, but don't jeopardize your health by not seeking the right help.

Be Consistent

We're all busy, and life is hectic. But take the two to three minutes needed each night to clean and moisturize your face. The skin care you invested in won't do any good sitting on the shelf in your bathroom. Take your makeup off as soon as you get home at night before getting too relaxed. Keep your moisturizer by your bed if that makes it easier for you to be faithful. You can't erase a wrinkle with a jar of cream but you can certainly defy the appearance of aging with a regular routine of good habits.

Makeover Action Plan: Instant Skin Makeover

This is a fun and easy minifacial that you can do today! Your skin will instantly look and feel better.

You will need:

A smashed-up banana **or** a smashed-up avocado

plus

A tablespoon of mayonnaise **or** a tablespoon of sour cream

- Pin hair completely off face.
- Wet skin with a warm, damp washcloth. Cleanse off makeup completely with your favorite skin cleanser or with plain or fruit-flavored yogurt.
- Rinse with warm water.
- Gently exfoliate skin on face and neck with your favorite skin scrub. (If you don't have one, make one by mixing a bit of sugar with enough margarine to make a paste. It works great, just be gentle.)
- Massage with fingertips for one minute.
- Rinse thoroughly with warm water.

- Smash the banana or avocado, and mix with a tablespoon of sour cream or mayonnaise.
- Apply with vegetable brush or fingers all over the face. Leave on for ten minutes.
- Rinse with warm water.
- Apply your favorite toner and nighttime moisturizer.

Now enjoy your velvety soft new skin!

SKIN CARE ACTIVITY

Organize your bathroom cabinet *today* so that taking care of your skin becomes a habit. Get rid of any old bottles of cleansers and moisturizers that you are not using. Make a shopping list of what you need, including cotton balls, Q-tips, washcloths, and so on. Once you've gotten everything you'll need, put the products on a shelf in the order that you will apply them. Being organized will help you stay true to your new skin care regimen.

12

The Magic of Makeup

"The best thing is to look natural, but it takes makeup to look natural."

—CALVIN KLEIN

"Uh, Mom . . . aren't you going to put on some makeup?" It was a Saturday morning, and my boys and I were headed out the door for a breakfast. Johnny, my eleven-year-old, was hinting that I should put on my more finished face. It has been three years since I started my new life and I must say, I have never felt better. My teenage boys have been amazed and appreciative of the change. I scooted off to the mirror with my makeup bag of tricks and in about six minutes I looked and felt 100 percent better. Johnny grinned, giving me a thumbs-up. I had finally crossed over from the low-maintenance frumpy mom to the mother my boys could be proud of. That is the magic of makeup.

Never underestimate the power of makeup. With every makeover I have created, the most beautiful changes happen with using a collection of pigments, paints, and powders that would fit in the palm of your hand. Every woman can achieve beauty and glamour with makeup. I will show you how and inspire you to be your own makeup artist.

"But I've never been the makeup type!"

If you think about it, none of us are born wearing makeup. Becoming the "makeup type" will be simple if you desire to look better and realize that makeup works magic.

"But I'm not very artistic!"

If you can draw a line with a pencil, you are talented enough to make yourself up with cosmetics. It's really simple. I will teach you step by step.

"I feel self-conscious and overdone when I put on makeup."

Remember the first time you wore a bra? Now that was a self-consciousness nightmare! The point is, you became adjusted to it! Have no fear. You will soon grow to love the way you look with makeup.

"Why should I have to wear makeup? Men don't have to!"

What a privilege to have the ability to change our looks instantly. Consider yourself fortunate.

"But I don't have time for makeup."

You can make yourself gorgeous in ten minutes, tops! That's faster than stopping at Starbucks for a cup of coffee. Don't let your custom-made java be more important than looking great.

Okay, enough cheerleading. You may already have makeup in your daily routine. Great. I hope you learn some new and exciting techniques in this chapter. If you are a makeup part-timer or a beginner, relax! I will start you off with easy, baby steps and gradually add additional, simple tricks. You can create your own routine that best suits your lifestyle and what you can handle. Making yourself up will soon become a daily habit and you'll become an expert at it. As you get better and faster at applying cosmetics, you won't view makeup as a chore or a mystery. It will be fun. Your makeup time will become a daily ritual—a gift of time you give yourself.

Makeup for Beginners

If you aren't the makeup type, don't despair. You are not alone! We don't come out of the womb wearing blush and mascara. Some girls rush into using cosmetics as soon as their parents allow them to. Other women don't start experimenting with makeup until they notice the first signs of aging. Makeup, after all, is not a requirement, it is a choice. You can choose what makeup you want to wear. Perhaps now that you've witnessed the makeovers in this book you are more willing to give it a try. Let's start you off with baby steps so that you can get used to feeling proficient at it. (If you are very comfortable with basic makeup application, go straight ahead to the detailed makeup lessons on pages 146–158.)

Essential First Steps: Lipstick and Mascara

The simplest and most essential first items to start using are lipstick and mascara. Adding color and shine to your lips and darkening and thickening your lashes will give you a more polished look in a matter of minutes. Practice applying just these two items.

Lipstick.
A basic lipstick in a twist-up tube is easy to apply.
- Choose a soft rose color slightly darker than your own lip color for a natural look.
- Glide the lipstick over your lips lightly and press lips together to blend.
- Once you've mastered this basic technique, you may step up to the lip lesson on page 153.

Mascara.

Nearly all mascara is dispensed by a brush applicator that comes with the tube. Higher-priced brands are not necessarily better than cheaper brands. The purpose of mascara is to darken the lashes, to thicken them, and to add body and shape.

- Choose dark brown if you are blond or red-headed, choose black if your hair is brunette or darker.
- Avoid waterproof formulations as they are difficult to remove. Use a water-resistant formula instead.
- Apply mascara lightly to bottom lashes first by holding the wand vertically and stroking lightly across the tips of the lashes. Pretend that the wand is a candle and the goal is to lightly singe the tips with your "candle flame."
- Next apply the mascara to the top lashes by first brushing downward on the topside of lashes. This will add thickness. Then brush the lashes up with the mascara wand to lift and separate the lashes.
- To make lashes extra thick, use a horizontal motion going back and forth between the corners of the eye to apply extra layers of mascara. You will know when to stop, when your lashes become difficult to comb.

Second Steps: Foundation and Blush

If you've never used foundation before, you may feel strange and pasty when you try it on. I encourage you to always apply at least a light coverage of foundation because a more even complexion will always look better and more youthful. Adding blush to the cheek area will eliminate the "monochromatic" look.

Foundation.

There are many types of foundation, from sticks to liquids. Take the time to go to a makeup counter that will allow you to try out many formulations and colors. You will know which is the right one for you. Go with your instincts. It's no more complicated than selecting paint for a wall in your home. Ask questions and decide for yourself.

- The most important consideration for selecting your foundation is that the color matches your skin exactly. Test the color on your jawline and let it set for at least one minute before evaluating. (Foundation tends to darken as it dries.)
- Apply foundation lightly over the entire face with your fingers or a cosmetic sponge, just as if you were applying lotion. It's that simple!
- Once you've tried this quick and easy approach to foundation, you may want to explore ways to add highlights and contours to your face. Go to the detailed foundation lesson on page 149.

Blush.

Blush is used to add a bit of color to your face and to add structure or a lift to the cheekbones. Once you've learned how, applying blush is so easy and takes only a few seconds.

- Select a powder blush in a compact that comes with its own applicator in a soft rose.
- Tap the brush applicator lightly on the surface of the powder, blow off the excess powder and stroke the brush gently over the cheekbone area a few times. Check yourself in the mirror. You should see a soft bit of color. Apply a bit more if needed.
- Now that you've learned this simple blush application, you may progress to a more sophisticated lesson on page 152.

First and Second Steps Review

Let's put together all the steps you've learned so far. Try the application in the following order:

1. Foundation
2. Mascara
3. Blush
4. Lipstick

After the foundation, apply the other cosmetics from the top of the face working downward to ensure that your hand doesn't disturb what you've already applied.

Great job! You've mastered the basics and are on your way to becoming your own makeup artist. I encourage you to apply makeup to yourself every day with these four steps. After a few tries, it should only take you two to three minutes to complete. Make it a regular habit even on your casual days. Do it for yourself, that important person you see every day in the mirror.

Intermediate Makeup

They say the eyes have it, and I wholeheartedly agree when you transform the eyes with a bit of shadow and liner. Adding drama to your eyes is easy when you learn the simple basics first before graduating to more complex techniques.

Eye shadow.

Shadows used to deepen and contour should be darker than your skin tone. Shadows used to highlight and bring the eyelid forward should be lighter than your skin coloring. In general, I recommend matte powder eye shadows.

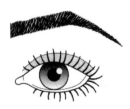

Figure 1

- Highlight the eyelid by simply stroking an oatmeal or beige shadow over the entire eyelid. This will bring the eyelid forward. See figure 1.
- Next, choose a neutral taupe/brown shadow for contouring the natural crease of the eye. Gently and lightly stroke a little dab

of shadow back and forth across the natural crease just above the eyelid. The goal is to add just a touch of shading to give you an almond contouring to the eye area. See figure 2.

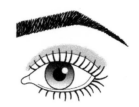

Figure 2

Now that you've tackled these two shadowing steps, adding a step or two more will be easy. For amazing and more alluring eyes, teach yourself how to give your eyes that extra drama with my eye makeup lesson on page 151.

Eyeliner.

Lining your eyes can be simple if you follow my logic: Line your eyes along the lash line to make the lashes look thicker!

- Make your line begin and end where your lashes begin and end.
- Make your line bolder where your lashes are longer.
- Taper your line as the lashes get shorter.
- Lightly sketch a soft line on the lower lashes with a basic brown pencil eyeliner. Holding your chin down and looking up at your mirror will make it easier and safe.
- Gaze down at your reflection as you lightly sketch along the top lashes.

Once you've got the hang of this eyeliner lesson, try experimenting with a liquid liner, or a cake eyeliner or dark shadow applied with a brush on the top lashes. The techniques for these are the same as with a pencil. There are no special tricks, just practice. I love the look of this style of eyeliner; see how it looks on Mary, see color insert.

Full Makeup Review

When putting together all the steps you've learned so far, the order of application will go like this:

1. Foundation
2. Eye shadow
3. Eyeliner
4. Mascara
5. Blush
6. Lipstick

Believe it or not, you've learned all the steps in putting on a great look. Certainly there is a whole world of makeup artists and techniques out there, but you should feel good about what you've accomplished so far. The best way to expand your own learning process with makeup is to practice. Good old trial and error is the name of the game. The way I look at it, any makeup when applied naturally is always an enhancement, so don't be fearful of making mistakes.

Becoming Your Own Makeup Artist

The next sections contain my top tricks for applying foundation, eye makeup, blush, and lip color. You may want to read and practice each page in sequence or jump around to the areas you need more help with. Have the book with you to refer to while applying and practicing each lesson. After practicing each lesson a few times, you will be a master at your makeup.

Tools

Makeup is easier to apply with sponges and brushes. Putting your makeup on is more fun when you have nifty tools at hand. Start by purchasing one nice brush at a time until you have a full set. For those on a budget, brushes are less expensive when purchased in a kit. Look for bargains at beauty supply stores rather than the department store makeup counter.

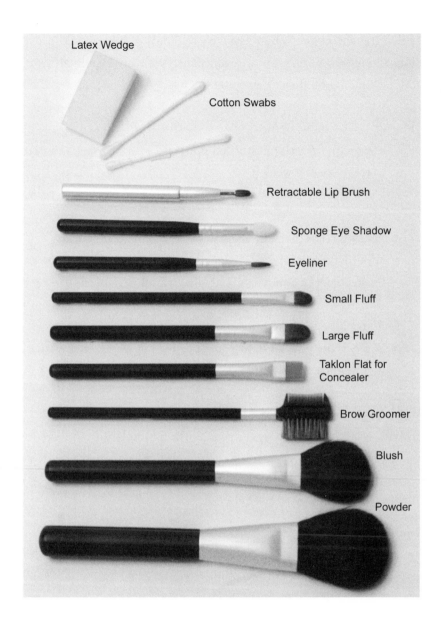

Latex Wedge

Cotton Swabs

Retractable Lip Brush

Sponge Eye Shadow

Eyeliner

Small Fluff

Large Fluff

Taklon Flat for Concealer

Brow Groomer

Blush

Powder

Foundation Lesson

I love applying colors to a perfect canvas, so I am a big fan of foundation. Foundation comes in dozens of formulas such as liquid, cream, powder, and pancake. Whatever formula you select, insist that the color matches perfectly. Avoid testing color on your hand. Instead, try it on your jawline, then wait a minute for it to set before evaluating the color. When applying foundation, you should use a latex sponge or a brush for an even, flawless finish. Apply all over your face including the eye area and the lips.

SIX TOP TRICKS FOR FABULOUS FOUNDATION

1. Start with smooth moisturized skin. Use a gentle exfoliator two to three times a week.
2. Use a creme-powder-type foundation for better coverage and to fill in pores.
3. Select a color that exactly matches the skin at the jawline.
4. When you're ready to advance, try using a makeup sponge or brush to apply foundation. It will look more natural, like real skin.
5. Blend all edges carefully—at the hairline, jawline, and neck.
6. Apply loose powder lightly and evenly, but avoid overpowdering. Skin should look moist, not dry.

ADVANCED FOUNDATION APPLICATION

For those of you who are comfortable using foundation and would like to go one step further, you have the ability to contour your fea-

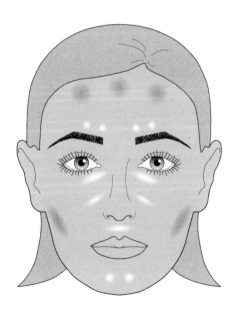

tures using two different shades of foundation. Referring to the diagram on page 150, apply the lighter shade on areas you want to highlight, and use the deeper shade on places you want to contour.

Eye Makeup Lesson

Playing up your eyes is easy if you understand where to place light colors (highlighting), and where to place deep colors (contouring). Colorful, sparkling shadows look great in the case, but don't always benefit your eyes. The idea is to make your eyes more vivid, not merely to display vivid makeup. I recommend three shadow shades for day or night. First apply a light color on the lid to highlight, followed by a medium shade to contour the crease. Finish with a dark shade to show off the lash line and smoke the deep outer corner of crease and eyelid. This technique will give you that smoldering smokey look you see on magazine covers. The placement of these three shades is the same for day or night. The color palette or depth of application is what changes the look. You can even use colors that coordinate with your wardrobe!

SIX TOP TRICKS FOR ALLURING EYES

1. Start with perfect brows, see page 154.
2. Apply foundation on your lids as a base for the smoothest shadow application.
3. Always use three colors of eye shadow—light, medium, and deep.
4. Use matte shadows for smoother-looking eyes, and to avoid telegraphing wrinkles. Add shimmering shadow lightly over lids and brow bone after matte application.
5. Always apply face powder lightly under eyes before applying mascara. It will keep the mascara from traveling and creating dark shadows under the eyes.
6. Apply the mascara in several layers for extra enhancement.

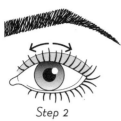

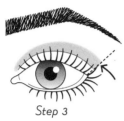

Step 2

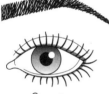

Step 3

Step 4

STEP-BY-STEP EYE MAKEUP APPLICATION

1. Start with foundation and powder on the eye area.
2. Start by applying a pale matte color on your entire eyelid. Pick a color that is lighter than your skin color.
3. The next step would be contouring the crease. Use a medium brown or taupe matte shadow to contour the crease. You should start at the outer corner of the eye and move toward the nose so that the shadow fades.
4. Shade the lash line by using a deep matte shadow starting at the outer corner moving toward the nose. The smudge line tapers as the lashes get shorter. (Apply shadow to the lash line on the top and bottom lashes.)
5. Apply the deep shadow on the outermost corner of the crease area and the outer third of the eyelid. Softly blend.
6. Finish with tons of mascara! Add false eyelashes for more flash!

Blush Lesson

Blushers add color to the face, no doubt, but their main purpose is to shape the face to give the appearance of higher cheekbones. That is why it is so important to place the blush application slightly under the cheekbone. It is ideal if the blush application gradually fades and gets lighter moving up to the cheekbone. Cream and gel blushers are on the market, but I use powdered blushers exclusively because I believe they are more user friendly in creating the fade. If you place a deep or bright color on the cheekbone or up near the eye, your cheekbone will look flat. Review these top tricks, then follow the step-by-step application for chic cheeks.

SIX TOP TRICKS FOR CHIC CHEEKS

1. Exfoliate skin two to three times a week for smooth cheeks. This makes for better blush application.

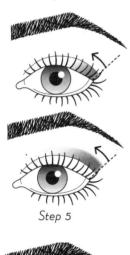

Step 5

Step 6

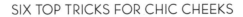

2. Get the right brush—full and supersoft for smoothest application.

3. For light blush application, powder cheeks first with face powder. For a richer-looking blush, apply directly after foundation, then lightly dust with face powder.

4. Use matte blush first in a medium to deep shade to contour under the cheekbone. Next apply a slightly shimmering blush at the top of the cheekbone.

5. Apply blush colors in a sweeping straight line. Don't make circles.

6. Blend and soften with an application of face powder or blend with a clean sponge.

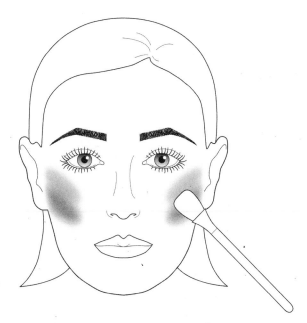

Lip Lesson

Lips should always appear soft and smooth, so skin care here is extremely important. Go for full lips; the fuller your lips, the better. You may use lip liner first to shape your lips or just use a lipstick and brush. If you choose to use liner for a barrier, make sure that you carry the lipstick over the liner. Bold lip liner looks unfinished. The shape of the upper lip is very important, so follow the steps!

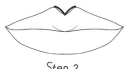

Step 2

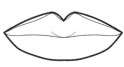

Step 3

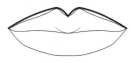

Step 4

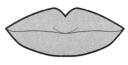

Step 5

1. Lips should be smooth and based with foundation or lip primer.
2. First line the "V" on the upper lip with lip liner, or lipstick and a brush. Arch your "V" slightly.
3. Connect the "V" to the corners of the upper lip. Use an arc instead of a straight line to make the lips appear full and round.
4. Line the lower lip from corner to corner.
5. Fill in with lipstick. Add gloss for extra shine.

SIX TOP TRICKS FOR LUSCIOUS LIPS

1. Keep lips soft and flake free. Exfoliate one to two times a week with a paste of baking soda and vegetable oil. Massage gently then rinse with warm water.
2. Moisturize nightly with AHA moisturizer.
3. Avoid drinking from straws. Think about it; the puckering when you suck from a straw makes the same lines as smoking.
4. Apply lip primer or foundation to make a smooth palette for lipstick.
5. For fuller lips use light medium colors, and add shimmer to the center of the upper and lower lip. To minimize large lips use deeper colors. Line lips slightly inside lip line.
6. For the longest-lasting lips, apply a long-wearing lipstick. Next apply a light application face powder followed by a bit more lipstick. For a shiny finish, apply gloss, but sparingly (gloss tends to break down long-lasting lipsticks).

Beautiful, Perfect Brows

Your brows are the most important feature of your face. Perfect brows will show off your eyes but overplucked, misshapen brows will detract from your look. Study the common brow mistakes, then give your brows a makeover by adding brow powder to replace missing hair.

The perfect eyebrow is easy to attain with tweezers and brow powder.

- The brows should start along an imaginary guideline that would be drawn from the nasal rim to the inside corner of the eye.
- The stem or base of the brow should be straight, not curved or arched. The thickness may vary but should be the same thickness from the start of the brow all the way to the apex. The line formed at the top of the stem should be parallel to the line formed at the bottom of the stem.
- The apex should never be flattened or removed with tweezing or waxing. The apex is the top peak of the brow. This peak is what gives the brow the lift. The apex is directly in line with the outer edge of each iris. Never thin out the brow until you reach the apex guideline.
- The end of the brow tail can be marked by the imaginary guideline that runs from the nasal rim to the outside corner of the eye.

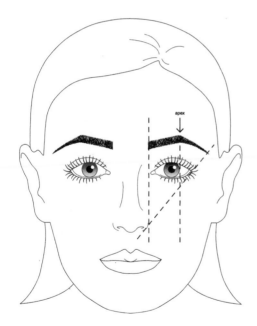

BROW MISTAKES AND CORRECTIONS

Commas.

Comma brows look like commas. The overall shape is too round. The bulbous stem was created by overtweezing hair prior to reaching the apex.

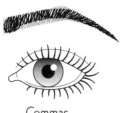

Commas

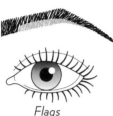

Flags

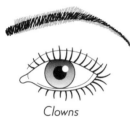

Clowns

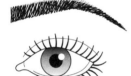

Flat Brows

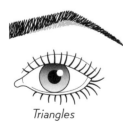

Triangles

CORRECTION FOR COMMAS: Reduce the thickness of the bulbous stem by tweezing from underneath in a straight line. Apply brow powder to replace missing hair below and above. Allow the missing hairs to return.

Flags.

Flag brows look like a flag on a flagpole. The brow stem starts out nice and straight, but the cleanout was done too quickly, leaving a long skinny tail.

CORRECTION FOR FLAGS: Correct with brow powder above and below the brow and allow hairs to return.

Clowns.

Clown brows make you look surprised all the time. If you raise your eyebrows in a real expression of surprise, the effect is worse. The hairs were tweezed out in a circle leaving no apex or lift.

CORRECTION FOR CLOWNS: Rebuild the straight brow shape with brow powder. Allow your brow hairs to return.

Flat Brows.

This happens when ambitious waxing is done to the top of the brow. Never take out hair anywhere near the apex. Flat brows will make the eyes look droopy and closed.

CORRECTION FOR FLAT BROWS: With a small brush, apply brow powder to build the apex.

Triangles.

The brow stem is tweezed at an angle on the way to the apex.

CORRECTION FOR TRIANGLES: Apply brow powder to brow stem to make stem thickness consistent.

SIX TOP TRICKS FOR BEAUTIFUL BROWS

1. It's all about shape. Study the shape you want before removing precious brow hairs. Don't overtweeze.

2. Trim long brow hairs.

3. Color gray brow hairs. Don't pluck them.

4. Use a brow wax instead of gel or clear mascara. It will hold brows in place without flaking.

5. If you've overtweezed, let the hairs grow. Stick to your desired shape and avoid tweezing hairs that are lonely. If you let them grow back, the lonely hairs will get a buddy soon and then you can help recover a shape with brow powder. Give them at least a year to recover.

6. Add missing brows with a matching brow powder. Use the powder just to replace missing hairs, but don't "chalk in" over existing hair to avoid heavy-looking brows.

STEP-BY-STEP GUIDE FOR BROW POWDER APPLICATION

1. Start with foundation and powder. Comb brows up with brow wax.

2. With a brush and brow powder, mark dots using an imaginary guideline. These dots mark the beginning, the end, and the apex of the eyebrow. See figure 1.

3. Using brow powder, fill in base of brow. See figure 2.

4. Fill in the brow from apex to tail. Keep the apex angular and strong. See figure 3.

Makeover Action Plan: Instant Makeovers Today!

Instant Makeover for Your Brows

Pin your hair completely off your face! Reread the eyebrow lesson on page 154.

Comb up your brows and set with clear mascara or gel. Trim the very tips with small cuticle scissors.

Mark your guide dots and build brow shape with brow powder.

After brows are filled in with powder, then tweeze strays with tweezers.

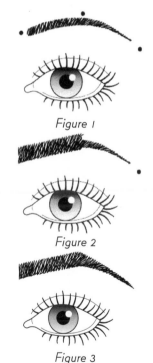

Figure 1

Figure 2

Figure 3

INSTANT MAKEOVER FOR YOUR LIPS

Remove all makeup with cleansing cream and warm water.

Mix a paste of baking soda and margarine. Gently massage over your lips for ten to thirty seconds.

This natural complex will remove dry skin from your lips.

Rinse with cool water and apply lip balm and/or moisturizer.

Refer to the lip lesson on page 153.

After applying a foundation around the mouth, practice outlining your lips with full guidelines; fill in with your favorite lip color and gloss to give your sweetie a kiss!

INSTANT MAKEOVER FOR YOUR EYES

Cleanse face with cleanser and warm water.

Trim and tweeze brows.

Treat your eyes to a softening exfoliating treatment. Mix a paste of baking soda and butter or margarine. Very gently massage the paste over the eyelid and under the eye while the eyes are closed. Remove with tissue followed by warm water and a washcloth.

Apply a lightweight moisturizer and foundation all over face, including the eyelids.

Refer to the eye makeup lesson on page 151. Apply the basic natural shadow application, followed by mascara.

Have a little more fun by layering some exotic shades over your daytime look. Call a friend and go out for the evening!

13

Beautiful Hair Every Day

"Gorgeous hair is the best revenge!"

—IVANA TRUMP

The phrase "bad hair day" is a reality with a lot of us now and again, but it doesn't have to be. Believe it or not, I find doing my own hair difficult and a bit frustrating. It's hard to co-ordinate the movements holding a brush and blow-dryer over my head. I can empathize with my clients and their hairstyling dilemmas. Like anything else, improvement comes with knowledge and practice.

Clients come to me often moaning about styling difficulties and looking to me for the magical, quick, and easy haircut. The problem is that "wash and wear" styles often look old-fashioned and frumpy. If I give in to these low-maintenance wishes, I fail as a beauty adviser. The trick is to create a winning style and teach clients the easiest way to achieve the look. Everybody wins.

Never believe that you can't style your hair. Twenty years ago, most of us couldn't operate a computer. We simply weren't good at it. As soon as it became evident that computers were vital to our lives, we learned real fast. You must decide that looking your best is key. I want you to receive a thousand compliments on how great you look because of your terrific hairstyle. No more getting by with that fast "out of bed and out the door" cut. You might as well get clipped at the barber!

As we progress through this chapter, keep reminding yourself that this is the new you who takes time for herself and is open-minded about learning how to achieve that new hairstyle.

Hair Types

Hair is like yarn; it comes in different colors, textures, and weights. Sometimes hair changes during the course of your lifetime. You may have started out with curly hair as a youth and found that it got straighter as an adult or vice versa. It is important to accept what kind of hair you have and try to work with it when choosing a style. Going "against the grain" often leads to damaged hair and unhappiness. For instance, you may choose to chemically straighten your very curly hair to fit today's smoother hairstyles. Next, you decide to highlight your hair for the streaky, blond look. Those two chemical actions together may severely damage your hair, leaving it dry and unmanagable. My best advice for hair that is naturally beautiful is to stay close to what you were born with. Slight variations in color or texture are fine in the hands of a good stylist. I will teach you how to safely change the texture of your own hair with some styling techniques and products.

Here is a list of terms to help you understand and determine your hair type:

Straight—Hair that does not have a wave or curl pattern.
Wavy—Hair that has a little bend or wave to it, not curly, but not completely straight.
Curly—Hair that has a definite curl pattern.
Fine—Refers to hair strands that are smaller than normal in diameter.

Medium—Refers to hair strands that are normal in diameter.

Coarse—Refers to hair that is larger than normal in diameter.

Wiry—Refers to hair that is coarse and somewhat unruly, such as gray hair.

Thin—Refers to hair that is less dense than normal.

Thick—Refers to hair that has a lot of density.

When examining your hair, you should be able to use three of these terms to describe your hair type. For example, my hair is wavy, thin, and fine. That translates to a head of hair that has a slight wave pattern. I have fewer strands than most people, and my hair shafts are very small in diameter.

Analyzing your own hair will help you understand the cut and style possibilities. You will make a better choice when selecting your ultimate haircut.

Choosing Your Hairstyle

Say yes to the style you really want—the style in your glamorous "new you" mind! Don't let that low-maintenance devil sitting on your shoulder talk you into an easy, frumpy style. Pick the look you want and I'll show you how to master it every day. My sources for inspiration and style shopping are the hair magazines found in the magazine section of the grocery or bookstore. More than a dozen publications come out monthly that are devoted to haircuts and styles. Pick the ones that feature well-known celebrities. Their styles are created by some of the most talented hairstylists. You can rest assured that you are choosing the latest looks that are fresh and glamorous. Purchasing a magazine before you go to a salon for a new style will give you a communication tool to help the stylist learn your personal taste.

Once you are in a hairstylist's chair, show him or her the styles that caught your eye. Ask the stylist if your hair type would lend itself to any of those styles. What your stylist says should help you narrow down the choices instantly. Once a decision has been reached and the cut is complete, pay close attention to what the stylist does to dry and finish the style. Ask questions and follow the styling technique step by step. Don't leave the salon until you feel confident that you can handle it at home. You can't be married to your hairstylist!

If possible, purchase the exact products and tools the stylist used to complete the hairstyle. Don't handicap yourself by leaving without the items you need. You are worth the investment. Leave-in conditioners, volumizers, pomades, and hair sprays are vitally important to create and hold the style.

Hopefully when you leave the salon, you will look and feel great with a fresh new style. Now it's up to you to keep it up on your own at home.

Shampooing and Conditioning

Keeping your hair clean and healthy is the first step in managing your hair. Most of us shower daily and for many people, this includes a daily shampoo of the hair. There is nothing wrong with cleansing the hair and scalp every day. The only drawback to the daily habit is having to style your hair every day. After working with hair for so many years, I have learned that most heads of hair stay clean for two to three days. Try to change your shampoo routine so that you are cleansing the hair every other or every third day. Styling your hair will be a more enjoyable experience if you don't have to tackle it daily.

The frequency with which you need to apply a conditioner will vary depending on the condition of your hair. Hair in a virgin state (meaning the hair has been unchanged by chemicals) may not even need a conditioner. If your hair is easy to comb out without tangling, then skip a conditioner. Normal or damaged hair that tangles easily requires a conditioning after every shampoo. Two types of conditioners work well. A rinse-out conditioner, which is used in the shower after you shampoo and rinsed away, should make hair easier to comb out but not leave a heavy buildup on the hair. A leave-in conditioner, however, is massaged into the hair after shampooing and left to dry. I love leave-in conditioners especially for hair that is dry or damaged. The hair will respond nicely to blow-drying and hot curling irons. Ask your hairstylist to select an appropriate conditioner for your hair. It is an important step to a successful style. It will keep your hair looking healthy and shiny.

Towel Drying

During the rest of this chapter I use the phrase "towel-dried hair." I really mean "towel-squeezed hair." Rubbing and drying the hair vigorously with a towel roughs up and damages the cuticle of the hair. A better habit is to squeeze the excess moisture out of the hair to prepare it for styling.

All the Right Tools

Having the right tools makes all the difference in the world when it comes to successful hairstyling, but you need only the tools that are appropriate for your hair. As a general rule of thumb, most styles can be achieved with a brush and a blow-dryer, a styling product, and a finishing product. Blow-drying can require two-handed coordination and is difficult for some people. Alternatives to blow-drying include using a curling iron, flat iron, rollers, and hot brushes. You may or may not know what all these tools are, so here's a quick overview to familiarize you with what's out on the market.

HARDWARE

BLOW-DRYER: A handheld gun-style dryer designed to dry hair quickly with fingers or a brush.

HOT BRUSH: A handheld, wand-style blow-dryer with a round brush attached. Hot brushes make it easier to dry and brush with one hand. Many clients find this much easier to use than a regular

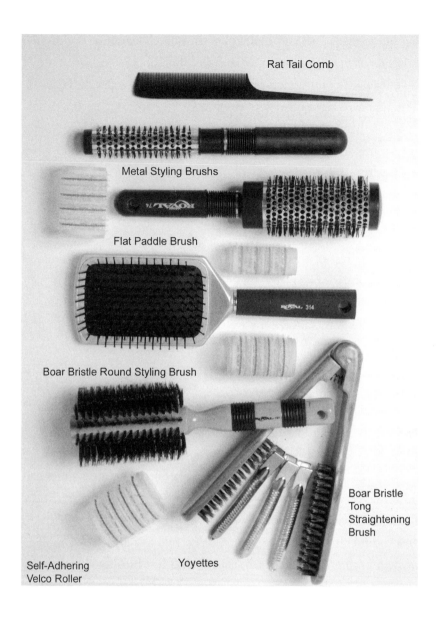

Rat Tail Comb

Metal Styling Brushs

Flat Paddle Brush

Boar Bristle Round Styling Brush

Boar Bristle Tong Straightening Brush

Self-Adhering Velco Roller

Yoyettes

blow-dryer. It is especially well suited for making curly hair smooth and straight. Look for one that has short bristles in the brush. Shorter bristles prevent tangling in the hair.

CURLING IRONS: A handheld round metal wand that heats up to curl or smooth the hair. Choose a clip iron rather than a marcel iron that hairstylists use. It will be easier to handle. Curling irons come in several diameters. To smooth and straighten hair, choose a larger one that measures one and a half inches. For making curls, choose a smaller one from five-eighths to three-fourths of an inch.

FLAT IRONS: A handheld iron with a paddle head used to iron out hair smooth and flat. They are great for making curly or kinky hair straight. Try to find one that has a temperature control. Flat irons are exceptionally hot, so avoid using them every day.

HOT ROLLERS: Rollers that heat up in a dry heat or steam unit. They come in many sizes. Choose a set that has medium to large rollers. Rollers can be very hot and should not be left in the hair a long time. The hair will become very dry from using hot rollers daily.

REGULAR ROLLERS: Rollers come in many sizes. Smooth rollers are made of plastic and require clippies to keep in place. I prefer self-adhering rollers, which are plastic rollers with a Velcro-type coating. They stay in place without clips and are very easy to use. For smooth and straight styles, select large rollers. For curly styles, use smaller rollers.

YOYETTES: Metal or plastic clips similar to clippies but longer in length. These are very important tools for dividing your hair into sections for blow-drying or using hot-styling tools. You will need up to ten, depending on how much hair you have.

CLAMP CLIPS: Plastic "jaw"-style clips that can also be used to divide the hair in sections. You will need four to eight of them depending on how thick your hair is.

LIQUID STYLING TOOLS

MOUSSE: A styling foam designed to give a lightweight hold and volume to the hair. Mousse is best suited for fine, lightweight hair to give shape, volume, and lift. Apply to towel-dried hair before styling.

GEL: A thick gelatinous substance designed to give a firmer hold to the hair. A good gel should not flake after it dries. Gels are usually used to give hair a wet look and are best suited for men or shorter hairstyles. Some gels are lighter weight and come in spray form. These are good for distributing throughout a thick or long head of hair.

CURL ENHANCERS: A liquid spray that aids the curl pattern in hair. These are beneficial to perk up a perm or curly hair. They should be applied to wet hair to help keep the integrity of the curl.

ROOT LIFTERS: A foam or liquid designed to lift the base of the hair off the scalp. These are fairly new on the market and aid tremendously in giving volume and thickness to thin, fine hair. They work so well to give lift, I recommend them over getting a permanent wave. Apply a root-lifting product to towel-dried hair before styling.

POMADES: These come in many forms, such as foams, waxes, sprays, and creams. They are designed to shine and polish the hair and to give texture and separation. The hardest decision to make is which one is best for your style. Ask your hairstylist to recommend the appropriate formula. Pomades are used on dry hair to finish the style.

HAIR SPRAY: A pump-type spritz or aerosol used to hold the hairstyle. Hair sprays are varied from light hold to firm. Just remember that the stronger the hold, the more alcohol is used, which can be drying. If you restyle your hair throughout the day, be sure to select a spray that is easy to comb out, so you don't break your hair.

My Secrets for Successful Hairstyling

To focus on how to style we're going to assume that you already have a new haircut and basically know what it should look like. My techniques are designed to achieve the desired look while saving time. If I can save you time, the task will be more enjoyable and you'll be more consistent about styling your hair.

BLOW-DRYING

Select your favorite styling product and work it into towel-dried hair. Comb the product through the hair to remove tangles and distribute the product evenly. Begin blow-drying your hair with your head upside down while standing or sitting. The idea is to dry the roots while the head is upside down. This will give the hair fullness and help create volume. You may lift the hair away from the scalp as you aim the dryer at the root area. Be sure to move the dryer around so that you don't heat up the scalp. Spend enough time in this position to get the hair 80 percent dry. It will make styling the rest of your hair easier.

Once your hair is nearly dry, stand up straight and set your dryer down. Now it's time to section your hair. Using yoyettes or clamp clips, section your hair into several layers. Start with the very top of the head and secure that hair section with a clip. The next layer is the temple section. You may section this part of the hair with two clips, one for each side. The third section includes the hair above the ears and to the back. Secure this with one clip. Now you should be left with a large section of hair hanging down the back. Divide this hair into top and bottom. Secure the top half with a clip, leaving the bottom half hanging down. Now you are ready to continue blow-drying with a brush in sections.

Using a brush in one hand and the blow-dryer in the other, finish drying the bottom section thoroughly. It should only take three or four passes of the brush and dryer to complete the section. You may choose to blow the hair turning under, flipping up, or just pulling the hair straight.

Set your dryer down and remove the clip from the top half of the back section. Proceed with dryer and brush. Dry this section thoroughly before removing the clip holding the next section. Finish drying the hair one section at a time, always from the bottom to the top. By breaking the hair up in smaller sections, the style is much easier to manage by yourself. You won't become frustrated with getting the brush stuck in your hair. Most important, by drying in sections, your hair will take on a better shape and the style will last longer throughout the day. Trying to dry your hair in one big section doesn't give the hair a chance to dry completely. If you quit styling when your hair is still damp, especially at the roots, the style will be incomplete or "poop out" in about an hour.

Once you've completed the top section, wait about one minute before putting the finishing products in. This will give the hair a chance to cool, which sets the style.

ALTERNATIVES TO BLOW-DRY STYLING

Blow-dry styling can be awkward for some individuals. If you have trouble operating a dryer and a brush, here are some other methods you can try.

HOT BRUSH: After drying your hair upside down until it is 80 percent dry, section your hair with clips, then proceed with a hot brush. This is a similar technique to the brush and blow-dryer, but many people find this method easier as there is no need to coordinate both hands. You'll still work in sections from the bottom up. Then proceed with finishing products.

ROLLERS: This is my favorite method and the one that I use personally on my hair. Blow-dry the hair upside down to get volume at the roots. Dry the hair this way completely. Stand up and while the hair is still warm, set the hair with self-adhering rollers. Spray the hair with a light holding hair spray and wait for about ten minutes. Take the rollers out gently so that you don't disturb the style, then continue with finishing products.

CURLING IRON: Blow-dry the hair upside down to achieve volume at the roots. After the hair is completely dry, divide and clip into sections. Work the curling iron through the hair one section at a time, starting with the bottom and working your way up. For a straight style, simply clamp the iron on the hair section and stroke the iron down the hair to smooth and straighten out the hair. To curl the hair, stroke each section first with the iron, then wind the hair around the iron and hold for only two or three seconds. Avoid the habit of baking the curl in with a hot iron, or you will dry your hair out.

FLAT IRONS: Follow the same procedure as explained in the curling-iron section above. Remember that flat irons are very hot and can dry out the hair. It is better to stroke the hair a few times quickly than to iron the hair very slowly. Using a leave-in conditioner will help to insulate the hair from hot irons.

HOT ROLLERS: The only drawback to hot rollers is that they get extremely hot and will dry out the hair if used with great frequency. Hot rollers tend to give the hair an old-fashioned look. If you use hot rollers, leave them in for no more than five minutes. Try a new styling technique if you are in a hot-roller rut.

DRYING CURLY HAIR

Curly hair is a blessing or a curse, depending on what you wish to do with it. If you have curly hair and want to wear it curly, then the styling game is easy. Staightening curly hair is a different story and requires a little more effort. Hair that is curly will respond better with a little extra conditioning. Try using a conditioner in the shower and a leave-in conditioner in tandem. The beauty of curly hair is that you can go longer in between shampoos.

Drying Curly Hair in a Curly Style.

You will need a blow-dryer with a diffuser and some clippies. A diffuser is an attachment for your blow-dryer that breaks up the force of the dryer to avoid blowing the curls around. It really helps keep the curl pattern consistent and prevents frizzing of the hair.

After applying a leave-in conditioner to wet hair, spray a liquid spray-gel all over and comb through with a wide-tooth comb. Using your hands, squeeze and scrunch the hair to form a curl pattern. The next step is a cool trick. It is designed to keep the hair curly up at the root area on top of the head where curls seem to drag out. The reason curls drop or flatten out at the scalp, especially with long hair, is because of gravity. When your hair is wet the water tends to travel down the hair, adding weight to the ends. This extra weight pulls downward and straightens out the curls at the top of the head. To prevent this, you need to take the weight off the curl pattern at the top. Using clippies, clip the hair in small sections at the top of the head one inch away from the scalp. The idea is to open the clip, place in the hair, and shove the hair up about a half inch toward the roots. You may use eight to ten clippies to accomplish this. As the hair dries, the initial curl at the base of the scalp will have a chance of surviving the weight of the wet, heavy hair.

Now proceed with drying the hair using the diffuser. You may bend over and hold your head upside down, letting the hair gather in the basket of the diffuser. Push up to further scrunch the curl pattern into the hair. Continue drying until the hair is 80 percent dry. I don't dry curly hair completely in order to limit the amount of frizzing. Don't forget to remove the clippies.

Drying Curly Hair in a Straight Style.

You will need to know how to section the hair with yoyettes. Please refer to the section in this chapter that explains the basic blow-drying technique. Before you start, it is important to give the hair the advantage of a product designed to straighten curly hair. Curl tamers are a more specific leave-in conditioner that you can get at a salon. Not only will a curl tamer aid in getting hair straight, it will keep the hair from curling up in humidity. Curl tamers make curly hair feel smoother and less frizzy. Put an abundant amount in wet hair, then section it before you blow-dry the hair in the upside-down method. Exceptionally curly hair needs to be straightened while it is still wet. If you try to partially dry it, then straighten it, you may not be as successful in removing the curl. Use a natural, boar-bristle brush that is round in shape. It will be the most effective in grabbing the hair to pull it straight. However, round brushes are notorious for getting stuck in the hair. A brush with short bristles will prevent this.

Proceed to straighten the hair one section at a time starting from the bottom and working your way up to the top. Straightening a curly head of hair requires patience. Once your hair is completely straight and dry, you may choose to make it even more sleek with a curling or flat iron. Be sure to resection the hair in clips before you go back through it with the iron. Because the straightening process is time-consuming, try to go two to three days in between shampoos.

Finishing Your Style

The biggest secret I can share with you to ensure that you look salon finished after styling your hair on your own is what I call the "Last Five Minutes" technique. Hairstylists deliver most of their magic in the last five minutes of styling. By the time you get finished with your blow-drying procedure, you may be tired of working with your hair. The secret to great-looking hair is to be patient for five more minutes to finish the look. This is when you should use a finishing product like a pomade to give an extra bit of texture and shine to the hair. A pomade helps to separate and detail the hair, giving more dimension and shape. At this point, it helps to use your fingers more than a comb or a brush. Have a picture from your look book handy as a visual aid. Don't give up until you like the way it looks. Use a light misting of hair spray to hold the finished style. Practice makes perfect, and you will get better each time you patiently work with your hair. If you are not getting the hang of it, call your stylist and ask if you can come in for some further styling hints. A good stylist will be more than happy to help you.

MORE HELPFUL HINTS

- Get regular hair trims or cuts even if you are trying to grow your hair long. Not trimming the hair in an effort to save length will cause ragged ends to break further.

- For healthy hair and hair growth, eat a well-balanced diet. Foods high in folic acid are beneficial for healthy hair growth.
- Beware of using rubber bands to tie back hair, as they tend to cause breakage. Use coated or fabric bands to prevent breakage. Remove them slowly and carefully.
- Never speed through the combing-out process, especially when your hair is wet. Damage and breakage to the hair are self-inflicted when we are in a hurry. Hair in a wet state is more fragile than you think. Use conditioner and detanglers to aid in combing the hair. Use a wide-tooth comb first, then a small-tooth comb or brush.
- If you have a dry or flaky scalp, brush the hair and scalp before shampooing with a natural boar-bristle brush. Many times a dry scalp simply needs to be exfoliated with a good brushing.
- To make hair shiny, rinse in ice-cold water. This can be somewhat uncomfortable, but you can rinse the hair, not the scalp. The cold water closes down the cuticle layer of the hair leaving it smooth and shiny.
- For oily hair or limp hair, avoid conditioning at the scalp. Conditioner can be applied just to the ends and midshaft.

Makeover Action Plan: Take Action Today

Make appointments for hairstyle consultations at two or three hair salons. The purpose of the appointment is to shop for a new stylist and to get some feedback on the possibilities for your new style.

BEAUTIFUL HAIR

Purchase a couple of hair magazines at the grocery or bookstore. Tear out the pages of styles that appeal to you. Add them to your look book. Don't be afraid to select anything that grabs your attention. Take these ideas to your appointments when you interview a new stylist. The pictures will help give you and the potential stylist some visual guidelines.

GET ORGANIZED TODAY

Strip down the drawers in your bathroom or dressing area to make way for your hairstyling station. Organize the area just like you would at a professional salon. Don't collect items that you are not going to use. Keep it simple and clean. Starting out with a great styling area will make the task of styling your hair easier and more fun.

14

The Cure for Your Closet

"Who said that clothes make a statement? What an understatement that was. Clothes never shut up."

—SUSAN BROWNMILLER

How would you like to give yourself an instant makeover in less than an hour? You can accomplish an immediate transformation by making over your closet. My closet cure is quick and easy and is based on one simple concept: *Get the guy out of your closet!*

I felt great after losing seventy-five pounds because my new shape made me look more like a woman. I had been wearing baggy men's clothing to disguise my fat, frumpy body. But there was a price to pay for a new slimmer physique. I had to buy a whole new wardrobe!

Looking back at photographs featuring the "old" Laura decked out in mannish loose clothing gave me an insight about my self-esteem. I was trying to hide a body that caused me embarrassment and discomfort. As I allowed my shape to go from one of a model to one of a frump I witnessed my wardrobe evolving from slender feminine garments to an odd array of oxford shirts, sweats, khakis, and Levi 501s.

Even the fly on my jeans was "male." I thought I was cool and hip. Sadly, I was not even remotely close to looking fashionable or cute. Instead I had made myself invisible. My unbalanced, chaotic lifestyle pitched me into a stupor and a daze when it came to selecting flattering clothes. Unconsciously I shopped for, or rather settled for, clothes to hide in. My attire was perfect if you lived in "Frumpsville." I was tired of living there. On the path back to beauty, I knew I had to toss out my old clothes along the way. I made a vow to dress like a woman again.

Denying Your Feminine Side

Once we left the 1950s, women stopped wearing bouffant hairstyles and dresses. At first, the freedom to wear pants like the guys was a thrilling experience of comfort and equality. Women did not have to be forced into stockings, high heels, and petticoats anymore. Liberated at last! I grew up during that time and found relief in the fact that I could stand up from the lunch table bench without the boys looking up my dress! At first, the switch to pants and jeans seemed like a positive political victory, similar to women achieving the right to vote. Lately, I'm not so sure, especially when you look around and view the way we dress today.

Genderless dressing has grown popular beyond wearing your brother's blue jeans. Designers like Calvin Klein and Abercrombie & Fitch keep pitching the androgynous styles at us year after year. They look great in a magazine ad, particularly if you are a seventeen-year-old supermodel weighing 115 pounds. For most of us over twenty-five years old, imitating this look can be a disaster. There is nothing flattering about throwing masculine clothing on a body that is ten to forty pounds overweight. If you add the casualness of the weekend (no makeup, wearing glasses, and a fresh out-of-bed hairstyle), you may not just be fashioned like a guy, you may be mistaken for one. (I was referred to as "sir" once in a hardware store by a young male clerk. I deserved it. My short blond hair and stout body clad in jeans and a polo shirt was reminiscent of a washed-up rock star.)

My message here is "Don't deny your feminine side." Take a stand and decide that you want to look like a woman, from head to toe, twenty-four hours a day, seven days a week. Be a woman, look like a woman, feel like a woman. This simple principle will give you a whole new outlook on the way you dress and style yourself. Everyone around you will take notice and react to it.

Get the Guy Out of Your Closet

I first wrote about my closet cure in my first book, *Natural Beauty: Pamper Yourself With Salon Secrets at Home*. Since then I have received hundreds of e-mails from women who "got the guy out of their closet," and they loved getting rid of him. These women wrote to me saying how they enjoyed their new, more feminine look and so did their men. Here's how it works: Go through your closet and dresser drawers. Hold up each item and say to yourself, "If my brother or boyfriend had this in his size, would he wear it?" If the answer is yes, get rid of it! I am suggesting that you throw out or donate to charity every single piece of clothing in your possession that a man would feel comfortable wearing. After this exercise, you may end up with only a few things to wear, like I did. That's okay. At least the clothes that you will wear from this point on will be contributing to your female beauty and not working against it.

I had three huge garbage bags of clothes for charity when I raided my closet. I was even wearing boxers for underwear. What was I thinking? If you are smiling at this moment, you are probably among the ranks of many women who let themselves be lured into casual comfortable clothing and believed that it looked okay. Right now, make a mental inventory of your wardrobe and plan a time when you can raid the closet. After that's finished, your mission will be to begin a plan to rebuild your wardrobe that will be more flattering and will declare that you are a beautiful, glamorous woman.

Girl Power

On your future shopping trips for a new wardrobe, make a pledge to yourself to seek and find the most feminine styles from head to toe. It's just as easy to purchase a pretty lacy bra as it is to buy the basic sports-type bra. Underwear can be comfortable as well as sexy; you just have to make a decision to pick the sexy styles. Sweats are not all the same. When buying workout wear, pick pieces that a guy would definitely *not* wear by selecting feminine colors such as pink or styles with bell bottom pants or halter tops. In every section of a clothing store, there is always a choice. Choose the feminine styles. Pass on the masculine goods. I guarantee you that immediately, shopping will be more fun and inspirational.

Create, Don't Collect

Women love to shop and buy clothing. It almost seems like a recreational event rather than just serving the functional needs of your wardrobe. Learn to create and build your wardrobe slowly and carefully. Avoid shopping just to collect multiples of the same garments. People around you don't keep up with your wardrobe or keep track of how many times a month you wear a particular outfit. You really don't need as many outfits as you may think. My strongest advice is to keep it simple with fewer ensembles. Know what you need to build on your current wardrobe before you even leave the house. This will keep you focused instead of buying impulsively, which leads to "collecting." A good policy for your closet is to only replace what you throw out. This will ensure that you keep the same number of garments on hand all the time.

Go for Quality, Not Quantity

It is better to buy one really great suit than a bunch of separates that are on sale. The one technique I admire that men employ with their wardrobe is that they invest in a few suits and rotate the shirts and ties. I have learned to spend more on a well-tailored jacket or suit that will float from season to season. The higher quality will speak mountains about your image and project your self-esteem. Trying to have dozens of ensembles that are of poorer quality just to wear something different every day will not serve you well. Keep it simple and tasteful.

The Perfect Fit

No matter what your size is, always be a stickler about having your clothes tailored or altered to fit properly. When shopping, ask the clerk if the alterations are included. If not, find a seamstress in your area who is proficient at alterations. Ill-fitting clothing will make you look frumpy and out-of-date.

Your Look Book

Back in chapter 3, I encouraged you to start collecting photos from magazines to create a personal portfolio or a look book. Your look should be well thought out before you go to the mall to shop for new clothes. Creating this portfolio of styles will help put your plan in motion. Flip through a fashion magazine and tear out the pages of clothing that appeal to you. You'll probably have many pages gathered, because you like the pants on one page, but the blazer on another page. You get the idea. Your look book will be your fashion plan you take to the mall. Your inner style may emerge very quickly. If so, it will be relatively easy for you to shop. If, however, you go through magazine after magazine and don't find anything that you like, try again in a few weeks. It may take a few tries to get your imagination going. You may be just a bit out of the fashion loop. Chances are that you are fearful or not yet in the mood to reoutfit yourself—if this is the case, don't go shopping! Wait until you get a better sense of how you want to look before squandering your money on a hodgepodge wardrobe.

Off to the Mall

I strongly recommend that you go shopping alone. You will be more successful in your mission if you can engage the help of store sales-people without the influence of a girlfriend, sisters, or mother. A shopping buddy's opinion may suggest you stay right where you are—in a rut. It also helps to know your budget before you venture out to spend. Fashion malls usually offer a variety of stores with many price ranges. Stick to the stores that fit your budget. Feeling good about your purchases will keep you smiling.

Ask for Help

With your look book in hand, march right up to the salesperson and ask for help. You are not doing yourself any favors when you dismiss a helpful clerk with that "just looking" declaration. The salesclerk usu-ally knows the inventory quite well and can assist you in wardrobe planning and future building. Show the clerk a page from your look book and watch them go to town putting an outfit together for you. A helpful salesperson will run for more sizes while you are in the dress-ing room. Learn to ask for his or her advice when it comes to defining your new look.

Display Your Best

If you're not the best at putting outfits together, you can put your best foot forward by copying the displays in the store. Look at store windows, the end aisle mannequins, and the display up on the walls for the hottest looks fresh out of the designer's showroom. When you see something that attracts your eye, consider yourself a smart fashion whiz, because that is exactly who put the elegant, tasteful, and complete outfit together. Most boutiques and stores hire artists, fashion experts, and display professionals to detail and coordinate displays. These presentations may be themed to the season and are loaded with terrific ideas. Simply select the same items in the display in your size. Voilà! Shopping made easy. It's almost like a "paint by number" lesson in fashion. Before I picked up on this little secret, I would spend hours sifting through rack after rack of garments, not finding what I wanted. Thanks to displays, shopping is fast and more fun.

Dress for Success

My suggestion here does not necessarily mean dressing for a profession. What I mean by "dress for success" is to think about what you are putting on every day, even on the weekends. Your image is everything that tells others who you are. Don't underestimate your wardrobe. When you feel and look good in the clothes you wear, you will project confidence every time. The right outfit can project your personal image and make a memorable first impression. If you are a stay-at-home mom, dress for yourself to please your sense of pride in caring for your home and children. If you work in a casual environment, don't dismiss the importance of your job, dress up just a little more than you need to. This will please you, and I bet you will perform better. If you work at the executive level or in a high-profile job, be consistent in your high-powered presentation but always be true to your femininity. After work, dress to enjoy your life with a sense of style. The right outfit can also help you demonstrate your romantic side.

Here are some things to look for while clothes shopping:

- Comfort
- Flattering fit
- Good color
- Right style
- Proper length
- Durable fabrics

Keep your shoes polished or washed. Have your best clothing dry-cleaned, and make sure everything is pressed and neat. Taking care of these details adds to your own sense of personal pride and well-being. It speaks once again to your own realization of your self-worth. If you believe in it, others will buy in to it. That's the dress-for-success philosophy I am talking about.

Your Closet Cure

You may need a day to cure your closet, or you may feel you are pretty much on track already. Whatever the case, don't put off the opportunity to give your closet a checkup. You can do it today. If you are projecting a weight loss soon because you desire a body makeover, get the guy out of your closet in the meantime. You may be left with only a few items, but you will start to look and feel better. As soon as you weed out the old clothes, begin a look book and a shopping plan. As your weight drops, get rid of the "fat" clothes. This will help you make the commitment to continue with a body makeover. Last, check your progress every once in a while by opening your drawers and closet and asking yourself, "Is this a woman's wardrobe or a man's?" The answer should be clear. Crystal clear. Have fun!

Makeover Action Plan: Cure Your Closet Today

INSTANT CLOSET MAKEOVER

This plan of action will show you how to lose weight. Lose the weight in your closet. How many items are destroying your feminine side? How many items do you have in your closet that are too small? Are you hoping to lose five to ten pounds so you can fit in them again? Whatever the reason, these clothes are clogging up your closet. Here is what to do:

1. Set aside everything that your brother, boyfriend, and or husband would wear if it were in his size. (Really scrutinize!)

2. Set aside all the clothes that don't fit perfectly. If nonperfect-fitting clothes can be altered, do so.
3. All the other set-asides should go to charity. Don't cry!

Now, take a deep breath and make a basic list of necessities. Chances are, you may want a body makeover, so limit your shopping at this time. Refer to your look book for the items that you will need. Make a shopping list. When you go shopping for clothes, look for a comfortable, flattering fit, a good color, the right style, the proper length, and a durable fabric. These clothes will last you a long time and you will love wearing them over and over again. Not to mention the compliments!

15

Beautiful Eating

"We are indeed much more than what we eat but what we eat can nevertheless help us to be much more than what we are."

— ADELLE DAVIS

You may not believe your body is beautiful yet, but it can be with a bit of effort. I use the phrase "beautiful eating" to encourage you to make the connection between what you eat and a beautiful body. The shape your body is in at this moment has everything to do with what you have fed it. If you are a regular fast-food eater, chances are your body shows it. I am guessing that many of you reading this book are overweight as I was, thanks to my daily diet of two to three meals served up at a drive-through. As I take you through my new style of nutrition, I encourage you to go back to basics and common sense when it comes to food. We tend to divert off this commonsense path when life gets busy and hectic. Since there is a fast-food restaurant on every corner in America, it can become a normal routine to "drive by" for an easy meal.

Common sense will tell you that regular meals of burgers and fries will kill any dream of having a pretty figure. Take a look around you.

Why Do You Think They Call It Junk Food?

There is no denying that America is faced with an epidemic of obesity. When I went to high school in the 1970s, fewer than a dozen students out of a thousand were overweight. At high schools around the country today, teenagers are getting larger and heavier. Sadly, there is a growing number of overweight and obese grade-school children as well. Why? It's not hard to figure out. Drive-throughs, fast food, junk food, so-called convenience foods, combined with computers, television, and not enough exercise. I know because I got caught up in the routine of going to work all day, dashing to day care to get the kids, then heading off to the drive-through for a meal and going home to crash on the couch. That's the biggest problem with fast food. It will put you on the couch. Why? Burgers, tacos, burritos, even chicken sandwiches, and especially fries and sodas trick you into feeling full, make you lethargic, and deplete your energy. You will feel satisfied, but your body will be sorely lacking the nutrition it needs. This fake "full" feeling leads us to believe we are properly fed after all, since we associate a full tummy with a good meal. The negative result is weight gain, sluggishness, slack muscles, even depression and fatigue.

I can't emphasize enough the importance of rejecting fast food. Today, I rarely let my children have a drive-through meal. We've made it a family policy, and remarkably everyone finds a much healthier way to fuel their bodies.

Why Diets Don't Work

My way of eating is not about dieting—I learned the hard way that diets don't work. One of the largest sections in a bookstore is dedicated to diet books. Hundreds of books have been written and marketed featuring the hottest new trick, plan, or idea on how to lose weight. The trouble with any diet is that eventually we revert back to eating normal food again, in some cases fast food or other poor food choices, and the weight returns. During my seven years of weight gain, I collected an entire shelf of the latest diet books looking for answers. You name it, I tried it—low carb, high carb, blood type diets, blood sugar diets, even the cabbage soup diet. My only gain besides more weight was a stack of hardbacks for the garage sale pile. You can't win the food game by stacking the deck with dieting tricks. The only way to get the body you've always wanted is to give your body what it wants and needs . . . nutritious, healthy food.

What Your Body Needs

Simply put, your body needs regular doses of highly nutritious food more often than you may think. Like many fitness experts, I stick to a plan of six meals a day rather than the traditional three. Most Americans continue to gain weight or fail to lose weight by overeating at these three meals. When you eat a large meal, your body can't use all the calories you consume, and eventually the surplus gets stored as fat. If you skip breakfast, starting your day with coffee or nothing at all, you are robbing your body of the most important meal of the day. Eating the first thing in the morning will give your body fuel and energy, and it will keep you from bingeing with a late morning donut and coffee or overeating at lunch. The key to looking and feeling great is to eat, not to starve.

The best fuel for your body is a balance of proteins, carbohydrates, vitamins, minerals, and some fats. The most harmful aspect of dieting is that many diets restrict you from eating the very items your body needs. For instance, the notion that your body doesn't need carbohydrates is just silly. Carbs give immediate energy and help regulate blood sugar. All you need to keep in mind is how many carbohydrates you should consume at a meal to fuel you with proper energy.

Like carbohydrates, not all fats are bad. Fats are needed for metabolism as well as keeping your skin, hair, and nails from getting dry.

The fats you need are found in fish like tuna and salmon as well as vegetable oils such as canola and safflower oil. Fats to avoid are saturated fats found in abundance at your local fast-food restaurant, in processed foods like chips, cookies, and margarine.

The big breakthrough in my personal nutrition makeover came when I learned about the importance of protein. Like many people, I was carbohydrate "addicted" and protein "starved" when it came to eating. When I was growing up, meat was considered expensive. Large families like mine stretched out the food dollar by creating a variety of ways to serve what amounted to lots of carbs. Casseroles were big in the 1950s and 1960s, giving way to high-carb addiction. Meals made up mostly of carbohydrates are often called comfort foods because they fill the tummy and make us feel good (like Mom's home cooking). The belly may feel good, but the results won't be good. Carbohydrates consumed without an equal amount of protein will eventually most likely be stored as fat. Protein not only helps to regulate blood sugar and energy metabolism, it supplies the amino acids and important nutrients for your muscle tissues. Feeding your muscles with protein is the first step to a more toned and sculpted body.

Vitamins and minerals are readily available every day in fresh fruits and vegetables. You may use vitamin supplements if you'd like, but make sure you research what you take with your doctor. Don't make the mistake of buying an array of bottles and putting together your own recipe. Supplements taken in the wrong proportion or combination are sometimes completely ineffective and can be harmful. I prefer to get the minerals and vitamins from fresh fruits and veggies, which also provide must-have fiber.

Dozens of products on the market claim they will burn your fat cells away, but I found that one of the best products is free—water. Lots of water. Water is necessary for decreasing fat and dozens of other body functions. Its intake will help flush out toxins from fat cells, which are stored in fat tissue and released into the bloodstream. The body will hold on to water if an adequate amount is not supplied. When you are dehydrated, your body excretes less water and bloating can set in. The National Research Council recommends at least nine cups of water a day for women (twelve for men). I find myself running to the restroom a little more often, but every time I do I remind myself, "It's in with the good and out with the bad."

Putting together the right combinations of food will not only help you begin to shed pounds, it will also boost your energy levels. After eating this way for just a few weeks, I was no longer a couch potato. My new way of eating allows me to keep up with my active boys and get to the gym every night with enthusiasm even after a long day at work. Try this new eating plan for a few days in a row and you'll feel a positive energy surge you will love. Here's how it works.

Feed Your Beautiful Body Routine

FOUR RULES FOR YOUR BEAUTIFUL BODY

- Consume six meals a day, six days a week.
- Each meal should consist of a protein and a carb.
- At three meals add a bonus vegetable or fruit.
- Once a week, take a day off; eat anything you want.

Before I explain all the details, I want you to understand that my beautiful body routine is not a temporary diet. It is a way of eating and fueling your body for the rest of your life. I have eaten this way successfully for three years and absolutely love it. Even with my busy and hectic lifestyle, I find it healthy, fun, and extremely rewarding. Initially, your body will respond with higher energy levels and weight loss. Eventually you will notice healthier-looking skin, hair, and nails and increased muscle tone.

EAT SIX TIMES SIX

Eating six times a day will keep your blood sugar level stable and give you the fuel you need to function. You should eat as soon as you wake up. I am not a breakfast eater so my wake-up meal is always a protein shake. After your wake-up meal, eat every two to three hours. This may go against your normal way of thinking but remember you will be eating smaller amounts of food at each meal. No more gorging on two meals a day. Trust me. The six-meal method will satisfy your hunger and help you reduce body fat. Eating more often keeps metabolism clicking at a higher rate so that you burn more calories constantly throughout the day.

PROTEIN/CARB COMBO

At each and every one of your six daily meals you should eat a portion of protein and a portion of carbohydrates. (See list on page 197.) The size of the portion is very important. Try to think of fitting the entire meal in your open hand. This portion size will be just right for your body. Bigger bodies or hands require a bit larger portions. I also measure in my mind by thinking of teacup-size portions. (Not coffee mugs!) Keep it small. Don't revert back to your old eating style of big sizes. The protein should be lean and fairly free of fat. Bacon and other pork products are not considered a lean protein.

BONUS VEGETABLE/FRUIT

At three of the five meals you can add an extra portion of fruit or vegetables from the selection list (page 197). Again, measure by imagining a teacup. Don't imitate crazy diets that steer you toward devouring huge plates of fruits or vegetables. Eating a lot of fruit doesn't necessarily melt off fat but *can* screw up your blood sugar level. Certain vegetables are too high in carbohydrates to aid in body fat reduction. Stick to the list. Watch out for the salad trap. Eating a huge salad loaded with extras and dressing can add up to huge calories. Don't let yourself be fooled at the salad bar. My old salad bar addiction caused me to gain a lot of weight. Never eat a fruit or vegetable alone, always with your protein/carb combo.

PROTEIN SHAKES

Protein shakes are perfectly wonderful to fulfill one or two of your meals a day. I had to use shakes because of my tight time schedule.

You can mix up the powdered kind in a blender or shaker, or create your own from scratch. Now you can even buy ready-made shakes in your supermarket that are great and relatively inexpensive. I have them in the trunk of my car and at work at all times. Look for shakes that have at least twenty-five grams of protein, and under ten grams of carbohydrates.

DAY OFF

That's right! One day a week you can relax and eat anything you want. The thinking here is that you will be better at staying on your routine if you are afforded a relief day. At first you may likely use this day to have fun and gorge on all the junk you've missed during the week. Eventually, you may learn as I did that overeating will kill your stomach and make you feel lousy. Now on my day off I rarely eat big meals. I enjoy eating rare foods like nachos or ice cream. Plan your day off each week to catch that special occasion of a party or wedding. Have a great time without feeling deprived.

THE PAYOFF

Sounds easy? It is! And guess what? You will be successful because you won't be starving, and you won't feel deprived. By giving your body regular meals of food packed with nutrients, your body will pay you back in spades. Your energy will soar, you will think more clearly, elevate your mood and emotions, and restore confidence and control. The funny thing about rescuing your body from junk food is that your health and energy improve so much that your cells will actually create cravings in the brain for more nutritious food. If you start to exercise regularly, your need for healthy foods will increase even more.

How to Get Started

Start right now! Go to your kitchen and open all the cupboards and the refrigerator. If you are really serious about changing your body and changing your life, you will toss out all of the items in your kitchen that are not on the list. If you live with other people, then try to section off their food from yours. Dedicate a shelf in the refrigerator and the pantry just for you. This will help you mentally separate your new healthy eating habits from others in your household who may not be ready for this change. Eventually, you may be able to get everyone in the family on the program.

Next, go to the store with this book for your shopping list. Don't worry about how to put the food together. Making complicated recipes isn't important. For the first few weeks, I want you to stick to the basic plan. On your very next meal in an hour or two, create a small meal from the list. You can make this happen today, not after you've read the whole book or in a week. Do it today.

Develop a Code

I don't mean a secret code but a code of ethics for your body. Mine is very strict. I want it that way because I love having the body I have now and never want to have my old frumpy, dumpy body back. Here's an example of Laura's Body Eating Code:

- I never eat at a drive-through or eat fast food.
- I never eat white bread, white rice, or regular tortillas.
- I don't do fancy coffee drinks (mochas, lattes, etc.).
- I don't eat donuts, pastries, or cookies.
- I don't eat candy (even chocolate).
- I never eat burgers, fries, tacos, etc.
- I don't eat fatty meat like bacon or pork.

I am as loyal to this list of don'ts as I am dedicated to not smoking or using heroin or cocaine. A client once asked me how I could avoid the temptation of chocolate. Well, it may sound far-fetched to some people but I believe that sweets that are not nutritious are just as bad and addicting as other vices that most of us would never partake of. If you set boundaries of saying no to cigarettes and drugs, then you can also say no to donuts and burgers. Certainly heroin is immensely more unhealthy for you than junk food or your daily mocha. But take a look around at how many Americans are overweight and obese, laden with depression and health problems. Addiction to food is killing people the same as drugs. I choose to say no to anything that is unhealthy for me and to food that will put me back in "Frump" prison. I choose to live by my code.

Give Yourself Time

I didn't develop this strict set of rules right away. I cheated a lot in the beginning and saw the weight increase and the energy decrease. I learned the hard way that it was ultimately better to be in control. As my body got leaner and stronger, I was deeply inspired to be good to myself and be loyal to my code.

Think about developing a code over the next few weeks and months that will strengthen the eating plan I've already laid out. You will have a place to write it down in the back of the book. You can choose to have a day off or not as I mentioned above. That is still your choice.

Dining Out

It's not hard to eat correctly at any restaurant if you follow my simple rule: Don't look at the menu unless it is your day off. Ask the waiter to prepare what you want from your list. Food establishments these days are flocking to provide the new low-carb meals. I have found that I can just ask for what I want, fresh and naked (without heavy sauces and side dishes) and the waiter won't look at me like I am nuts. Be specific. Grilled, not fried. No sauces. No heavy dressings. No extras.

Drive-Through Emergency

If you get stuck with no other choice but a fast-food restaurant, I have a few suggestions that may help you stay on target. It requires a little creativity and some basic items you can keep in your car. (I am assuming that if you are hitting the fast-food restaurant, you are doing so because you are on the go.) You will need a collection of small packets of soy sauce, vinegar, mustard, and a bag of whole-wheat pita (pocket) bread. I'm not crazy, we always have a bag of pita bread when we are running around town. My kids eat it plain for a snack. I keep it for junk food emergencies.

- Order a chicken salad without dressing. Ask for some lemon wedges and some pepper. Slip the salad into the pita. Add mustard, soy, lemon, or vinegar. You'll love it and it will fill you up.
- Order a grilled chicken sandwich without mayonnaise or sauce. Ask for extra tomato and lettuce. Discard the bun or bread and slip the chicken and garnishes into a pita. Season as you like.
- Order two plain hamburgers (not supersized); hold the secret sauce or mayo. Ask for extra tomato and lettuce/onions and eat in the pita.
- At Mexican fast-food restaurants, the only idea I have for you is to order chicken tacos with extra veggies and serve in the pita or steak/chicken fajitas following the same routine.

The secret weapon to fight junk food temptation is your whole-wheat pita. They taste great and fill you up while eliminating fried or greasy foods from the meal. It's a cinch to create a variety of healthy meals on the road. Just because you find yourself very busy or on the run, don't settle for a junk food meal. Use your common sense and eat what's healthy. Throw away what is not. *Don't just eat it because it's there.* Remember, there is a fast-food restaurant on nearly every corner in America. If you make them your fueling station and continue to put fast food into your body, your body will be their best advertisement.

Guest Relations

It's tough sometimes to stick to a healthy eating plan when you are an invited guest at someone's home. Be creative and polite. I don't explain why I eat the way I do; I just take portions of what is on my list and avoid the rest. When a hostess tries to coax me to have a helping of fried chicken, I take it but don't eat the skin. No big deal. If it's your day off, have fun.

Meals at Work

Some of the clients I counsel on food have mentioned the problem of eating so many meals at work when they don't officially get a break. I prepare my "work" meals ahead of time, usually on Sunday afternoon, and keep them in Ziploc bags. Since the meals are smaller, it only takes ten minutes to eat. The most important thing is to stay on your program, even if you are grabbing a quick protein shake to sip at your desk.

Food for Thought

Our bodies are amazing machines, finely tuned and functioning every minute of every day. The food your body needs should be thought of as fuel first and foremost. Enjoying the food you eat is one of the pleasures of life. In time, you will get pleasure from fueling your body the right way. You will receive rewards and pleasure from the way your body looks, the way it functions better, and the increased energy you will experience. Diving into a slice of chocolate cake or devouring a juicy double cheeseburger may deliver momentary satisfaction, but I've found there is nothing more delightful than glancing in the mirror and seeing a trim and fit reflection of yourself. As you embark on your body makeover, try to see the big picture. A beautiful body is awaiting you as soon as you make the choice to reveal it. Celebrate yourself with healthy food because your body deserves it. Bon appétit!

Makeover Action Plan: Raid Your Kitchen Today

A HEALTHY NEW START

Make over your kitchen to give yourself a fresh start with your new beautiful eating plan. Reread pages 189–191.

- Get rid of all processed or canned food except for light/fat-free mayonnaise, soy sauce, vinegars, mustards, light/fat-free dressings and seasonings.
- Get rid of all snacks, junk food, and sweets in the pantry, refrigerator, or freezer.

Say good-bye to what you thought was healthy, like white rice, white bread, and breakfast cereals with sugar.

SHOP FOR BEAUTIFUL FOOD TODAY!

Go to your favorite grocery store with the food list on page 197.

- Stay on the perimeter of the grocery store.
- Fruits: Berries, apples, oranges, peaches, bananas.
- Vegetables: Potatoes, sweet potatoes, spinach, broccoli, tomatoes, carrots, lettuce, cauliflower, celery, cucumbers, squash, green beans, asparagus, cabbage, and mushrooms.
- Dairy: Low-fat yogurt, low-fat cottage cheese, eggs or egg substitutes.
- Bakery: Whole-wheat bread/bagels/pita/buns.
- Aisles: Vinegars, low-fat dressings, canola or safflower oil, seasoning and spices, soy sauce, canned tuna in water, brown rice, barley, oatmeal, and whole wheat pasta.

PLAN REMINDER

Write down or copy the following plan outline three times. Keep one list in your wallet, one in your office, and one at home. Soon your new way of beautiful eating will be a way of life.

Six meals a day, six days a week

Each meal = protein/carb

At half the meals add a bonus veggie

Eight glasses of water a day

One day a week = day off = eat anything

GOOD NUTRITIOUS FOOD LIST

PROTEINS	CARBS	BONUS VEGGIES AND FRUITS
chicken breast	apples	apples
crab	barley	artichoke
egg whites or substitutes	beans	asparagus
ground turkey/chicken	brown/wild rice	broccoli
lean ground beef	corn	brussels sprouts
lean ham	low-fat yogurt	cabbage
lobster	melon	carrots
low-fat cottage cheese	oatmeal	cauliflower
round/sirloin steak	oranges	celery
salmon	whole wheat pasta	cucumber
swordfish	peaches	grapes
shrimp	potatoes	green beans
tuna	squash	green peppers
turkey breast	strawberries	lettuce
	sweet potatoes	melon
	whole-wheat bread, etc.	mushroom
		onion
		oranges
		peaches
		peas
		spinach
		strawberries
		tomatoes
		zucchini

Note: There are fruits on both the carb list and the bonus list. That's fine, just don't duplicate at a meal.

PROGRESS REPORT
Name:
Date:

	DAY 1		DAY 2		DAY 3
Meal 1		Meal 1		Meal 1	
A.M.		A.M.		A.M.	
P.M.		P.M.		P.M.	
Meal 2		Meal 2		Meal 2	
A.M.		A.M.		A.M.	
P.M.		P.M.		P.M.	
Meal 3		Meal 3		Meal 3	
A.M.		A.M.		A.M.	
P.M.		P.M.		P.M.	
Meal 4		Meal 4		Meal 4	
A.M.		A.M.		A.M.	
P.M.		P.M.		P.M.	
Meal 5		Meal 5		Meal 5	
A.M.		A.M.		A.M.	
P.M.		P.M.		P.M.	
Meal 6		Meal 6		Meal 6	
A.M.		A.M.		A.M.	
P.M.		P.M.		P.M.	

	DAY 4		DAY 5		DAY 6
Meal 1		Meal 1		Meal 1	
A.M.		A.M.		A.M.	
P.M.		P.M.		P.M.	
Meal 2		Meal 2		Meal 2	
A.M.		A.M.		A.M.	
P.M.		P.M.		P.M.	
Meal 3		Meal 3		Meal 3	
A.M.		A.M.		A.M.	
P.M.		P.M.		P.M.	

DAY 4		DAY 5		DAY 6	
Meal 4		Meal 4		Meal 4	
A.M.		A.M.		A.M.	
P.M.		P.M.		P.M.	
Meal 5		Meal 5		Meal 5	
A.M.		A.M.		A.M.	
P.M.		P.M.		P.M.	
Meal 6		Meal 6		Meal 6	
A.M.		A.M.		A.M.	
P.M.		P.M.		P.M.	
DAY 7—DAY OFF—ENJOY A TREAT!					

Write a Code of Ethics for your body (see Laura's Code on page 192):

1. _____

2. _____

3. _____

4. _____

5. _____

6. _____

7. _____

Make three copies—keep one on your refrigerator, one in your wallet, and one on the dashboard of your car.

16

Beautiful Body Fitness

"Over the years our bodies become walking autobiographies, telling friends and strangers alike the minor and major stresses of our lives."

— MARILYN FERGUSON

When people compliment me on my figure these days, I appreciate it and often smile because I remember all too well how dreadful, unshapely, and slovenly my physique was just a few years ago. Like the Cheshire Cat hiding a secret, I grin inside, holding back my words, "You should have seen me when I was 194 pounds just a few years ago!" I reshaped my body in my midforties, so I believe that you can, too.

Before you heave a heavy sigh or roll your eyes at the thought of exercise, let me reassure you that building a beautiful body is a lot easier than you may think. The plan I have in store for you will surprise you with its simplicity. The key to success in building a beautiful figure is to work out in a highly effective manner and to be consistent. If you apply these two factors, you will have a beautiful physique— it's only a matter of time. How much time? That depends on what condition your body is in right now. Don't worry. You can make great changes at any age.

You have already read several stories about women just like you who tapped in to their own self-motivation and accomplished some impressive body transformations. The common factor with each and every woman was that she had a lightbulb moment, then made the commitment to change. That was the tough part. Once the decision was made, carrying out her fitness plan was simply a matter of dedicating time each day to get the workout in. I hope you've made the decision to take action toward beautiful body fitness. I will share with you my approach to trimming off extra pounds and sculpting your muscles for a body you will be proud of.

Same Body, Different Day

Guess what? My body, your body, and everyone's body is the same body we are born with. The human body changes because of positive influences, neglect, or abuse. The most important truth I learned during my transformation was that the human body is amazing in its adaptability. It responds wholeheartedly to any and every influence, condition, and force to which it is exposed. For instance, if you eat well instead of putting junk in your mouth, you will have more energy and feel better. If you exercise, your muscles will get tighter. If you do nothing but lie around every day on the couch, your muscles will soften and atrophy, making you feel lousy.

Your beautiful body is already a part of you. You may be soft and flabby from lack of exercise or overweight from overeating. Once you deplete the excess fat and strengthen the soft muscles, your body's beauty will be revealed. Think about this—everything you will need for that beautiful figure is already in your body: blood, veins, bones, muscles, and so on. It's all there. All you have to do is feed your body the right food and manipulate your muscle tissue to grow a certain way with body movement. It really is that simple. Once I came to this realization, I was filled with enthusiasm. It was as if there were seeds planted in my flowerbed and all I had to do was add the water and fertilizer and clear out the weeds. If I followed all the steps, I could enjoy beautiful flowers in my garden.

Dump the Excuses

When asked "How did you lose all that weight and get in shape?" I am happy to respond in the interest of helping other women. Most often I am halted with a series of excuses such as the following.

"My metabolism is slower than other people's."
Everybody has a slower metabolism when they don't exercise. Exercising regularly is the key to boosting your metabolism.

"It's hard to lose weight as you get older."
Your body will respond to good nutrition and fitness at any age. We just have a tendency to lose interest in ourselves as we get older and life gets busy.

"I don't have time to work out."
Remember, we all have the same amount of time. Think of the big picture: if you are fit, you will have more energy to get other tasks done faster.

"I'm too tired after work to go to the gym."
Yes, a friend of mine coined the phrase "Reentry is hell!" But if you could just dedicate yourself to going to the gym for just one week, your newfound energy will take over from there.

"My whole family is heavy, we're genetically fat!"
Be the first one in your family to change! Although genetics is a factor with some individuals' abilities to gain or lose weight, don't give up on trying to eat better and become more fit.

"I've ruined my body and I'll never get it back."

Wrong! No matter what shape your body is in now, you can always improve it in appearance and health.

That's the whole point of this chapter. *Your body can and will improve immediately when you take some simple steps toward change.* The first step you have just read about is to feed your body better food. The next step is to start developing your muscles so that your body will take shape and gain strength. Last, you need to lower your percentage of body fat to expose your newly sculpted muscles.

Make an agreement with yourself to dump the excuses! If you hold on to them, you will stay the way you are.

Building Muscle Tissue

My secret to reshaping my body and losing seventy-five pounds was predominantly due to weight lifting. When I share this secret with people who ask about my weight loss, I always receive feedback opposing weight lifting. Women in general seem to have formed a lot of misconceptions about weight training when, in fact, most women I have talked with have never really tried or learned how to properly lift weights. It is by far the most efficient way to develop a trim and firm physique in a relatively short amount of time. You will not get bulky and huge, I promise! By lifting weights, your body fat will be reduced. Here's how it works.

When you lift a heavy weight, in essence what you are doing is stressing the fiber in the muscle that is lifting and lowering the weight. Over the next twenty-four to forty-eight hours, the muscle fibers grow and repair themselves. Your entire body will start to get tighter and be more shapely as this repair process occurs.

Chewing the Fat

Here's the exciting part. As your muscle fiber repairs itself, it requires energy to get the job done. This extra energy will be supplied from your stored body fat, provided you don't overeat. Think of your muscles like an army that requires a source of energy. When you work out your muscles, the army gets bigger during recovery. This larger army requires more food so it will eat up your storage of body fat (again, if you do not overeat). Within just a few weeks of weight lifting, you will feel your clothes getting looser, not tighter. I can tell you from experience that you will be amazed at how quickly your body will register progress.

Personally Train Yourself

I believe that most of us are shy about weight lifting because we don't know how to lift or how to use the equipment. That may be why people stick to the same old piece of equipment and do not get the desired results. I admit I was intimidated to use anything but a stair-climber until I read a book about weight lifting that featured photographs of women lifting free weights. Free weights are dumbbell-type weights, not machines. I took that book to the family gym with me and slowly went through each move step-by-step until I memorized a routine. Within a week, I no longer needed the book. Once I mastered the movements, I was no longer shy about using the weight floor.

What about a personal trainer? I have nothing against hiring a personal trainer except that you may become dependent on him or her for motivation. Personal trainers can show you how to lift the weights but they can't lift them for you. If you can't afford a trainer, don't worry. You can afford to check out a library book or buy a book on training with weights.

Member of the Club

Do you have to join a gym? Of course not, but I will tell you that my gym time is very precious to me. I am fortunate to live where there is a terrific family gym that has a children's section, making it a dream for all of us to go together. It is what I do with my boys nightly instead of watching TV. Our membership is less expensive than buying a mocha a day at Starbucks. We fit it into our budget.

The really great thing about joining a gym is that you can usually receive free training and help. Another positive factor is the inspiration of seeing other adults of all ages working out and taking care of themselves.

Women have remarked to me that they feel intimidated about going to the gym when they are out of shape or they don't want to work out at a gym where there are men. (On a lighter note, I find it amusing that we women don't mind sitting in a salon with men around while our head is loaded up with tinfoil and crazy hair colors!) I can understand the intimidation factor, but remember that the gym is there to help you get in shape. Everybody there is pretty much in the same boat, all desiring to get or keep a healthy physique. Wear baggy, loose clothing and go for it! I admire the people I see every day at my gym, especially the larger folks who are struggling to get started. I say, "Good for you!" As far as working out in a gym with the guys around, all I can say is that I have learned a lot by watching the weight-lifting techniques of men as well as women. I've found that most people in the gym are focused on what they are doing in their own workout and are far too busy to look at me. Try not to let intimidation stand in your way of going to a good gym, although if this truly bothers you, there are gyms that cater only to women. Find a fitness center that is very near to your home with a wide range of operating hours.

Home Gym

If joining a gym is out of the question, don't despair. You can create a great workout area in a corner of your home. All you need is a collection of dumbbells in various weights and a simple workout bench that can convert from flat to incline. They have nice affordable systems at many fitness stores and even superstores like Wal-Mart and Target. Start out first purchasing the bench and a set of five- and eight-pound dumbbells. In the next several weeks, you can purchase more dumbbell sets of ten, twelve, fifteen, and twenty pounds. It took a year for me to advance past twenty-pound sets, so trust me when I caution you to not overbuy in the beginning.

Weight Lifting for Dummies

This will be easy, so please don't feel like a dummy if you are a novice at lifting weights! Weight lifting is a very smart way to exercise. You will see and feel results faster than with any other form of exercise. Once you master your routine, you will enjoy the sense of accomplishment from it.

One of the basic forms of weight lifting is something you do every day when you raise up on your toes. Your calves are lifting your body weight! Now think of the beautifully developed calves of a dancer! That should give you an idea of the results one can get from weight lifting.

There are two movements when lifting a weight. *Concentric* is when you lift the weight. *Eccentric* is when you lower the weight. It is very important to think of these two actions as equal in the amount of energy spent. Always lift and lower the weight slowly and deliberately with good form. Many people make the mistake of going too fast in a swinging or pumping manner. You will get done faster, but your muscles will not respond as well. Lifting weights is not an aerobic exercise. Going faster will not produce better results.

The Secret's in the Spaghetti

The purpose of lifting and lowering a weight is to create fatigue in the muscles. This fatigue and stress in the muscles will create a stimulation in muscle fiber growth and repair. To achieve results, you must work out a muscle until it nearly expires or feels like spaghetti. The first time I worked out with weights the right way, I could hardly lift my arms up on the steering wheel to drive home. When I got home to take a shower, it was equally as difficult to lift my arms and adjust the showerhead.

If you have worked out with weights or machines before and failed to experience "spaghetti" arms or legs, you were probably lifting far too little weight. A lot of women cling to the myth that toning and firming is best accomplished by using light weights but lifting a lot of repetitions. Believe me, this arm-flapping method will do nothing but waste time. To get results—to get those beautifully toned, tight upper arms and tight, round tush—you must reach the spaghetti stage! To experience this, you must lift a weight heavy enough to completely exhaust your muscles after a routine of lifts. You can design a routine for yourself using sets of reps.

Sets and Reps

Sets and reps (repetitions) are basic vocabulary words for weight lifters. A rep is a complete cycle of lifting and lowering the weight. Many people perform ten reps to exhaust the muscle, then rest. These ten reps make up a set. For beginners lifting weights for the first time, I recommend slow deliberate movements and performing three sets of ten reps resting in between each set.

Be a Heavy Weight

Remember to use a heavy amount of weight to exhaust the muscle you are working out. At first, determining the amount of weight will be a guessing game. Let's imagine you are curling your biceps with two individual dumbbells. Start with a five-pound dumbbell in each hand. As you lift and lower slowly, count to yourself, **one.** Keep lifting and lowering slowly until you get to the count of five. The fifth lift should start to get difficult. If the fifth is so easy that your arms are flapping, you need to start the next set with a heavier dumbbell. By the time you get to lift number ten, you should be quivering as you lift. You should barely be able to finish the lift. Feeling "quivers" at ten is the secret to how much weight you should be lifting.

Take a Minute

In between each set of reps, you should wait one full minute doing absolutely nothing but focusing on the next set. Your muscles need to rest for sixty seconds before starting the next set.

Muscle Groups

Divide your workout into upper body muscle groups and lower body muscle groups. On day one, work out chest, arms, and shoulders and abdominals. On day two, work out the legs, buttocks, and calves. For each muscle group, perform two exercises. For instance, if you are working out your biceps on your upper body day, perform two different exercises that work the biceps muscle. For each of these two exercises, you will perform three sets of ten reps. The whole point of weight lifting is to completely exhaust your muscle to the point of feeling limp. Go for spaghetti. It's not about sweating or huffing and puffing.

Remember to rest from weight-lifting sessions for each muscle group for at least forty-eight hours. This is why I suggest you alternate working out your upper and lower body—it allows the muscles to recover. The resting period for a muscle is just as important as the workout.

You Design Your Own Weight-Lifting Routine

You can design your own upper body routine! Simply look through the photographs in a weight-lifting book or magazine and select two exercises that work the following muscle groups.

- Chest
- Deltoids (shoulders)
- Biceps
- Triceps
- Abdominals

You can actually cut out photos and assemble them in a book to take with you to the gym. Do the same for your lower body routine:

- Gluteus maximus, or "glutes" (buttocks)
- Quadriceps, or "quads" (front thighs)
- Hamstrings (backs of thighs)
- Calves

As you work out each muscle group with a specific exercise, remember to perform three sets of ten reps, resting one minute in between each set. Your weight routine should be mastered before adding aerobics in order to learn the correct form and movements. Your weight routine should alternate days, for instance Monday/Wednesday/Friday or Tuesday/Thursday/Saturday. Remember, you get to enjoy a day off.

- Start with the upper body only your first week.
- Lower body only the second week.
- Alternate upper and lower body the third week and continue alternating weight workouts.

During this first three-week learning stage, simply take a walk on the days you rest from weight lifting. Walk for at least ten minutes but not more than thirty. This will prepare you for adding in aerobics with your weight routine. If you are feeling energetic, walk briskly. Your first three weeks getting into a fitness plan allow you to focus on learning a weight-lifting routine and making it a habit. Then you'll be ready to really get moving with aerobics!

Aerobics—A Matter of the Heart

Can you imagine getting a beautiful body without having to huff and puff for hours and hours? Most people believe that aerobic exercise such as jogging or stair-climbing for an hour or more is the best exercise you can do. That is a myth. Aerobic exercise and getting your heart rate up is good for your heart and lungs as well as circulation, but the good effects can be achieved in smaller doses. I encourage only eighteen-minute aerobic sessions after a three-minute warm-up. The beauty of this aerobic plan is that it can be easily accomplished even if you've sat on the couch for the last several years. You can get your aerobic exercise at the gym or outdoors. Choose anything you want as long as it raises your heart rate. (My favorite is speed walking on an incline treadmill.) If you are an avid runner, go for jogging or running. Other great methods for aerobics are rowing, spinning (bicycling), elliptical jogging, and stair-climbing.

I know that you may be doubting me right now—I was skeptical as well. For seven years I put in at least three or four hours a week on a stair-climber and consistently gained weight. The more I gained, the harder I pumped, sweated, and later collapsed breathless on the couch. I wasn't getting results. You may have experienced the same thing. When you overdo aerobics, your body becomes exhausted, loses energy, and can even burn your muscle tissue instead of fat.

The reason we believe that long sessions of aerobics will get results is because it seems logical that breathing hard and sweating for an hour will "burn" fat. It's true that aerobics will consume energy, but the most effective fat burning happens when muscle fibers grow and recover. That is why I want you to try to build your muscles with weight lifting and sprinkle in aerobics in between weight workouts. You will burn more fat in a shorter amount of time and will absolutely love your body's response.

Only Eighteen Minutes?

Yep! Your aerobics workout will be a cinch, especially if you start working into it gradually (outlined in the Makeover Action Plan at the end of this chapter). Each workout will begin with a casual three-minute warm-up, making no real effort except to get your body moving. The eighteen-minute session should take you through three phases of six minutes each. After your warm-up, begin your first six minutes by putting forth a basic level of energy; we'll call this level one. If you are a jogger, this would be a medium-paced jog. At level one you should feel yourself breathing deeply. After six minutes at level one, pick up the pace and increase the effort. Your breathing should quicken. This is level two. Try to hold the pace for the full six minutes. Now you are twelve minutes into your workout. For the last six minutes you will be at level three, and I want you to really push yourself. Exercising at this higher intensity will bring you better results than a medium pace for a longer duration. High-intensity aerobics in short spans of time are fabulous for burning fat.

Adding in Aerobics to Your Weight Routine

After three weeks of mastering your weight-lifting routine, simply replace your walk with an aerobics session. On your first aerobics day, start with an easy three-minute warm-up, then try to complete the entire eighteen minutes of aerobics. Use your common sense when creating your three levels of intensity. Obviously if you haven't been doing any aerobic exercise in years, you will only be able to handle walking briskly. That's the beauty of this intensity climbing method. You adjust it to challenge your own body. As you continue from week to week, you will increase the pace as your heart and lungs get stronger.

Empty Tummy Bonus

It doesn't matter if you choose to work out in the morning or the evening; however, working out on an empty stomach will bring you faster results when it comes to reducing body fat. Another factor in fat reduction is to avoid eating for one hour after working out. Your body will continue to burn calories and fat for hours after you exercise. Postexercise meals should be lean and small. Remember the teacup method!

Putting It All Together

Here's a sample of what your schedule should look like:

Monday—Weight-lifting upper body
Tuesday—Aerobics
Wednesday—Weight-lifting lower body
Thursday—Aerobics
Friday—Weight-lifting upper body
Saturday—Aerobics
Sunday—Day off

Note that when you start all over again, you will start with weight-lifting the lower body. If you follow a simple routine of weight lifting and aerobics and use the techniques for beautiful eating, you will feel more energetic, optimistic, and hopeful about your health and well-being. The added bonus is that your body will look better within weeks!

To Infinity and Beyond

The reason so many people give up on exercise is because they think it is a temporary fix, like an instant diet. It isn't. The only way you will be truly successful at revealing your beautiful body is to understand that fitness is as necessary and vital as eating and breathing every day. Most of us wouldn't think of going to bed without brushing our teeth. If we neglect our teeth, they will eventually fall out. Adapt the same code or regulation for your body. Don't go to bed without working out. Your body will fall apart if you don't take care of it. Your body is as precious as your teeth. Start gearing your thinking to taking care of your body for the rest of your life.

Beyond the Physical

I confess that when I first started weight lifting, I was interested in looking better. What I didn't know then that I know now is that my workouts are equally beneficial for my mind. Now when I go to the gym for my workout I spend thirty to forty-five minutes not just for exercise but for mental and emotional balance. I tune out the rest of the world and focus strictly on the accomplishment of moving those weights up and down, or reaching that eighteen-minute mark on the clock. When I leave, I feel confident that I accomplished my goal for the day and that I gave myself a gift of time and good health. Try to think of your workout as a privilege, a gift, and a blessing of self-improvement rather than "having to exercise."

Your body will give you what you ask for. Be a friend to your body. It is going to be with you for the rest of your life.

ADVANCING TO TEN—NINE—EIGHT

Once you've mastered lifting with the basic routine of three sets of ten reps, you can step up to a more advanced routine I call 10—9—8. Here's how it goes:

> Lift ten reps so you get the quivers on the tenth lift. Rest a minute.
> Add more weight and lift nine reps. Rest again for a minute.
> Add even more weight for eight more reps.

You should have spaghetti by now. If not, start with more weight at the beginning of the set.

Makeover Action Plan: Beautiful Body Fitness

DESIGN YOUR WEIGHT-LIFTING ROUTINE

Don't *wait* to talk yourself in to "weights." Get a weight-lifting book or magazine *today* and start making a small book of exercises by stapling the pictures together. Divide the pages into two sections, upper body and lower body. This booklet should be small so you can take it to the gym with you.

Use the chart on the next page to log your actual workouts. You may want to make photocopies of this chart to keep track of your progress.

FIND A GYM

Call around town and scan the newspapers for the prices of local gyms. Make appointments to tour at least two fitness centers!

SHOP FOR FITNESS

If you can afford it, buy a pair of weight-lifting gloves and an outfit to work out in. If you choose new shoes, you may want to choose red ones—your very own ruby slippers.

MOVE YOUR BODY TODAY!

Go for a ten-minute walk. Enjoy the outdoors! Your goal on this walk is to simply get moving for those precious ten minutes. If you want to walk longer, fine.

Jump Start Fitness Plan

- Week One   Weight routine for upper body
                  Walk ten minutes each day
- Week Two   Weight routine for lower body
                  Walk ten minutes each day
- Week Three   Alternate upper & lower body routine
                  Walk ten minutes each day
- Week Four   Alternate weight lifting with aerobics

Beautiful Body Fitness Log
Progress Report
Name:
Date:

DAY 1	DAY 2	DAY 3
Exercise	Exercise	Exercise

DAY 4	DAY 5	DAY 6
Exercise	Exercise	Exercise

STEP SIX

Living Your Dream

"Only I can change my life. No one can do it for me."

—CAROL BURNETT

17

Your Dream, Your Choice

"Goals are dreams with deadlines."

—Diana Hunt

By now you have read about many other women—real people just like you who felt somewhat lost or depressed. Life's challenges gobbled them up and buried them with responsibility. Some of these women felt just a bit out of the loop while others were truly suffering and in despair. By introducing them to the concept of self-love and self-caring, they found a renewed sense of hope in their lives. Life made sense again, and they felt in control.

The big question is why? How can a new hairstyle or losing fifty pounds have such a profound effect on one's outlook on life? Well, it's not the new haircut or makeup change that solves life's problems. The secret is realizing your self-worth and embracing it. When we treat ourselves with pride and expend the same amount of effort for ourselves as we do for others, we feel fulfilled, satisfied, and content. When we give ourselves permission to go to the gym, try a new hairstyle, and make over our appearance, we benefit from the compliments; more important, we reap the emotional rewards from the efforts we make to care for ourselves.

My makeover friends have been remarkable inspirations. As you end this book, I share their words of joy, which put everything in perspective:

Susan, a fifty-year-old mother of two, wanted to look and feel as glamorous as she did when she was in the entertainment business at twenty. "I'm going to have lip gloss on when I take my last breath, and it will probably be hot pink."

—Susan McFerson

Colleen woke up one day and hated how she looked in a family video. She couldn't hold her head up in public and that was a crushing blow. In the course of one day, she mustered up all the determination she had and took action. "My message to anyone who reads this book is to change everything. It is a total lifestyle change."

—Colleen Morgan

For Mary, life had suddenly dealt her cards from the responsibility deck. Taking care of everyone else in her family seemed to be her lot in life. With an attitude adjustment, Mary changed her thinking and carved out a chunk of time for herself each day. She learned that you can't be of service to those around you unless you have the energy that comes from taking care of yourself. "I'm giving myself permission to have my own hobbies and spend time doing totally frivolous things that I would have never done before."

—Mary Pierce

Stacey felt trapped in a rut believing that girls should wear long hair. At her new executive-level job, she knew she looked like a girl, not like an executive. She decided to take control and go for a change. "My new look makes me feel more confident, polished, and presentable. I've noticed a big difference in how clients perceive me."

—Stacey Ward

As long as Kerry was involved in a relationship, she made an effort to keep herself up. When the relationships ended, she found herself spiraling downward. After her final epiphany Kerry chose to change her life for herself, not a guy! Taking the position that her self-image is more important than the image she presents to others gave Kerry the drive to control her life. "I feel confident. It's easier to deal with stress because I feel good about myself."

—Kerry Davis

Kellene chose to have a makeover because she saw the amazing results of a coworker's transformation. Little did she know that her makeover would have such a profound effect on the way she perceived life. The power of beauty ignited a spark in Kellene's life. "Before I would crumble and fall apart when something in my life changed. Now, I let the little things roll off my back and I am better equipped to handle the big stresses."

—Kellene Kozub

Like many of us, Heather felt that her sole purpose in life was to micromanage her children's lives. But suddenly she realized that being a walking incubator and full-time nanny drained her love of life. Heather decided to take charge and restore the balance of being a woman as well as a mother. "Getting my priorities in order meant taking care of myself. Being a single mom, I realized I had to be a healthy role model for my kids."

—Heather Fries

Barbara taught high school and was firmly entrenched in the belief system that it shouldn't matter what you look like. After her makeover she felt the power of the compliments from others around her who noticed her radiance. Suddenly the philosophical teacher beamed with a new, outgoing personality. "I am much more approachable to other people now."

—Barbara Arrowsmith

Many people spend their lives doing things for other people but neglecting their own desires. Are you spinning your wheels every day accomplishing task after task but doing nothing for your own personal benefit? In many cases the loss of balance in our lives is due to loss of control of our life. It's time to take control.

It's easy to blame others for our unhappiness. In reality, we are the ones who make the ultimate decision on how our lives will be spent. Your life right now is the result of your decisions. If you feel worn out, overworked, or just plain lazy, do something about it. Nobody else will do it for you. Make the decision to be good to yourself and to feel good about it.

Living Your Dream

In a nutshell, you can live the life that you want. I believe that you can have it all; be a wife, a mother, a professional and also be an individual and a woman. If you give yourself permission to enjoy being a woman, you will be a very successful wife, friend, mother, boss, and coworker. You can and should take care of yourself. It's your right to be beautiful and glamorous and feel good about it.

The bottom line of my message in this book is that what we experience in our lives is a result of the choices we make.

Step 6, "Living Your Dream," is the final step toward the new you. You must take that step on your own. Nobody can do it for you. If you are ready to treat yourself with the same care and kindness as you give to everyone around you, begin your transformation. If you have not started your Makeover Action Plan at the end of each chapter, start today by reviewing each chapter and spending the time with yourself filling out the exercises and activities. Each and every step is an important move toward living your dream, the life you've always wanted with confidence, hope, and optimism.

If you have completed all of the Makeover Action Plan activities and exercises then you are well on your way to A Beautiful New You. The success of your transformation is now in your hands driven by your heart, your desire, and your intelligence, what you've learned with this book. Have courage on your quest to embrace the beautiful changes. As you receive compliments and encouragements from coworkers and friends, share with them your glorious story and please tell them about this book.

I wish I could be by your side to cheerlead for you and witness your new image, your new outlook, and your new life. I will be with you in spirit and invite you to keep notes and photographs on your progress. I welcome your highlights of your journey via e-mail at laura@lauradupriest.com. Congratulations!

INDEX

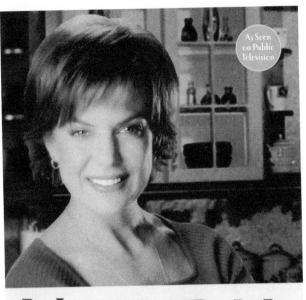